THE BEST
BABY
NAMES
for GIRLS

EMILY LARSON

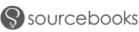 sourcebooks

This publication is designed to provide accurate and authoritative information in regard to the subject matter covered. It is sold with the understanding that the publisher is not engaged in rendering legal, accounting, or other professional service. If legal advice or other expert assistance is required, the services of a competent professional person should be sought.—*From a Declaration of Principles Jointly Adopted by a Committee of the American Bar Association and a Committee of Publishers and Associations*

Published by Sourcebooks
P.O. Box 4410, Naperville, Illinois 60567-4410
(630) 961-3900
sourcebooks.com

Library of Congress Cataloging-in-Publication Data

Names: Larson, Emily, author.
Title: The best baby names for girls / Emily Larson.
Description: Naperville, IL : Sourcebooks, 2019.
Identifiers: LCCN 2019008404 | (trade pbk. : alk. paper)
Subjects: LCSH: Feminine names--Dictionaries. | Names, Personal--Dictionaries.
Classification: LCC CS2369 .L37 2019 | DDC 929.4/403--dc23 LC record available at https://lccn.loc.gov/2019008404

Printed and bound in the United States of America.
SB 10 9 8 7 6 5 4 3 2 1

Contents

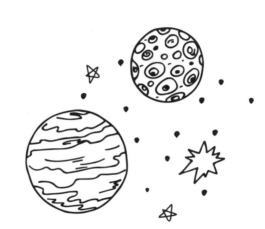

Introduction

Congratulations, you're having a little girl! And now that you've discovered the gender (or even if you haven't yet and are just hoping!) it's now time to buckle down and sift through the countless options available to you until you find the perfect name! But where do you even begin? Girls' names can be tricky, and the options (and opinions) are endless. As if preparing for the arrival of a baby isn't stressful enough, you are now under the added pressure of giving your child a name that she will have to live with for the rest of her life. Add to that the never-ending suggestions from well-meaning family and friends—and possibly a few arguments with your partner—and baby naming can become quite the daunting task! But it doesn't have to be. Believe it or not, you can actually have fun with the baby-naming process, and this book is here to help. Why browse through a massive compendium of baby names (half of which won't even apply to your child!) when you can breeze through *The Best Baby*

Names for Girls and discover the perfect option for your family? And even if you've gone through all of the lists and still haven't found the perfect fit, advice and journaling prompts appear throughout to help guide you to discovering the perfect little girl name for *your* family.

Yes, names influence first impressions. Yes, names sometimes spawn not-so-flattering nicknames that can follow a person all the way through retirement. Yes, names affect children's self-esteem. Yes, names are often obligatory ties to family. And yes, there are thousands to choose from. But what you must keep in mind is that this decision is yours. If you choose a name you take great pride in, your child will be proud of her name as well.

Of course, choosing a name requires some forethought— and therefore work—on your part. Even if you've had a name picked out since you were six years old, it is still a good idea to look around. Your child might not be all too appreciative of the fact that ten baby dolls (and possibly several pets) before her carried the same name. Besides, tastes change. Just as the thought of eating broccoli turned your stomach when you were a child and now it's your favorite vegetable, that name you had chosen so long ago may now leave a bad taste in your mouth.

Parents find several different ways to begin the baby-naming process. To some, it is important to incorporate a family name, so this becomes their starting point. To others, religion is a major factor in choosing a name. Some prefer to seek out a meaning or virtue, while others simply want a name that sounds good. What it all boils down to is what is important to you. So, before you begin scouring these pages, making endless lists within our journaling prompts, and seeking the advice of others, be sure to determine what it is that you want from a name.

The following chapters offer advice, tips, and suggestions to help you maneuver the baby-naming maze for your future daughter, and hopefully have a little fun along the way. Follow a few simple guidelines, keep your mind open, save your humorous and cutesy titles for your pets, and your baby will have a name she is proud to hear, say, and write forever.

Above all, remember that the decision is yours and you are going to find the perfect fit for your little girl.

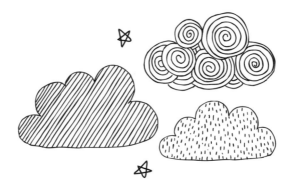

How to Choose
a Baby Name

P arents often find that the most challenging aspect of choosing a name is knowing where to begin. Let's face it: your kid has to live with the name you choose *forever*. (Or at least until she's old enough to legally change it herself.) To get going on your list, write down names you have always liked. Was there someone in school whose name you secretly wished you had? Did your favorite soap opera or sitcom have a character with a cool, trendy name? Browse the names chapters of this book and use the journaling prompts to jot down any that stand out (or names you think of along the way). Perhaps you are already receiving suggestions from friends and family. Are there any that appeal to you? List all the names you can think of that have caught your attention (in a good way) and list any family names you'd consider using.

Once you have a few (or maybe a few sheets' worth), consider the following attributes and see how each measures up.

Popularity: Past, Present, and Future

Every year yields a new crop of trendy names that makes last year's list, well, outdated. While these fresh, fun names are fabulous and exciting, they also face the threat of being "so five minutes ago." Of course, there are those names that have always been and always will be popular; they're classic and chic, and they always make top-ten lists. They're the names that are trendy one minute, but still sound good thirty years from now. The key to giving your child a popular name that he or she can be proud of is to avoid trend traps altogether, such as movie-character names or TV-icon names that have a popularity shelf life of about six months. Often, a child named after a memorable television personality will always be linked with that person's TV character or personality traits.

One factor that makes a name popular is variation of spelling on a familiar or common name. While the new look might be pleasing to the eye, it might become a nuisance when you (and eventually your child) have to constantly correct others, telling them that Denice is spelled with a *c*, not an *s*. Similarly, if you're looking for an exceptionally rare name, you'll constantly be correcting both the spelling and the pronunciation.

At best, name trends give your child individualism. At worst, they ostracize him or her from a society of "regular" names. However, more and more parents are creating their own names or choosing from a more eclectic list of foreign names, vintage names, surnames, and place names. And since the unique-name pool is rapidly growing, chances are that your child's classmates will have unique names too.

The increasing popularity of foreign names allows parents to honor their families' cultures and give their children a sense of heritage. Irish, Scottish, and Welsh names are on the rise, while Celtic boys' names for girls (Brynn, for example) have become popular. Greek, Russian, and Italian names have more presence than they did years ago, as names like Kaitlyn and Tatiana become more visible.

A recent revival of names like Millie, Alice, and Agnes give a new perspective on some old favorites. While these names might seem classic or old-fashioned to us now, most of them were the trendy names of their time. During a period when a respectful tip of the hat was greeted by a graceful curtsy, these names reflected the chivalry and ladylike charm that made up society back then.

The use of surnames is another trend that seems to appear in cycles. Names like Madison, Palmer, Kennedy, Mackenzie, Taylor, Jackson, and Spencer can all be used for little girls. What's more, surnames can prove to be a convenient alternative to using the first name of a family member you'd like to honor. If you want to use a surname for your daughter but are afraid that it sounds too masculine, spell it in full on her birth certificate and legal documents, but shorten it for everyday use. For example, if you love the name Jackson and want to use it to honor your great uncle, call your child Jackie for short.

Meaning

A fun, creative, and often unique way to choose your child's name is to look for positive associations that come with the name. It also makes the naming process intentional and more special. If one of your favorite places is a wooded area where your family vacations once a year, look for names that have "trees" or "earthy" in their meanings. You can also look for names that reflect your favorite color, time of year, season, animal, art, character trait, and flower. If your favorite relative loves to visit Ireland every year, and you wish to honor him or her, choose an Irish name for your baby and use your relative's name for the middle name.

It's a good idea to look up the meaning of the names you've put on your list because the last thing you want is to frighten your child if she finds out her name means "unlucky in life." A name should evoke good feelings, positive thoughts, and pride. It should also be significant to you and your partner. Meanings are a way for your child to feel connected to you, to your family, and to life. Of course, if you like a name just because, that's okay too.

Family Names

Using family names to create your child's name is a wonderful way to pay tribute to loved ones. Additionally, if after five hours you're still staring at a blank piece of paper, jot down all the names of your family members, including grandparents, aunts, uncles, close cousins, or even close friends of the family.

What do you do if your late grandfather's name, Jerome, just isn't appealing to you, but you still want to include his name in your little girls'? The way around that is to us a variation instead, like Romey. And if you'd love to honor your grandmother, but Dorothy feels a bit too old-fashioned for your daughter's first name, how about adding it as her middle name or using a variation like Dot or Thea? The intent is still there, the name is more appealing, and the family is happy.

List some important family members and friends. Are there any names (or variations) here that you'd like to use for your little one?

....

....

....

....

....

....

....

....

....

....

Origin/Ancestry

Perhaps you want your daughter's name to indicate her heritage. After all, it's an important part of her identity, and connecting with it only adds to the richness of her character. Similarly, if you come from a particular religious background, you might want to explore that group of names too. If your family has been following a tradition for many generations, such as naming first-born children after saints, but you have a different name in mind, consider moving the traditional name to the middle. You'll make your family happy and still get to use the name you want.

If you and your partner come from different backgrounds, selecting one name from each to create the first and middle names is a great way to compromise. If you're still having issues over whose name goes first, make them both part of the first name and use a hyphen. As for whose name goes before the hyphen, pick one out of a hat and be done with it. Julie-Ana is a combination of French and Spanish names, and in this case, the hyphen can be removed to spell Juliana.

A family tree and history can be helpful resources when linking your baby's name with your heritage. For example, if your grandparents' ancestors come from a village in France where they operated a cheese business that had been passed on from generation to generation, the name Monterey would be fitting. Or, if there were many carpenters in the family, Cedar would be appropriate for your little girl.

Spelling and Pronunciation

While creative spellings and pronunciations of traditional names make a name unique, some parents can go a little crazy with it. The more difficult you make your child's name to spell and/or pronounce, the more annoying it becomes for them to constantly correct people.

Even if the name is as clear as Robin, but spelled Robbynn, your daughter will still have to spell it out every time someone writes it down because they will undoubtedly spell it traditionally. The following list provides examples of how a small change can have big impact on a name.

- Replace *i* or *e* with *y*: Bryttany, Eryka, Karyn, Krysten, Kym, Lauryn, Maryssa, Mysty.
- Add an extra letter (*h* or silent *e*): Alissah, Annah, Donnah, Lisah, Mariah, Shaye, Taylore.
- Replace *s* with *z*: Alexzandrea, Izabelle, Izadore, Jazmin, Louize, Roze, Suzan.
- Add to or take away from double consonants: Britany, Coleen, Jenifer, Jesica, Marilynne, Nanncy, Sarrah, Sheri.
- Add a capital letter in the middle: AnnaBelle, DaKota, JulieAna, LoraLai, MaryAnne, McKenzie, MoNique.

Stick to one change per name. Too many different styles make the name look like the parents were trying too hard to be different. Once you narrow your list of names down to the top contenders, play around with different spellings to see how each one looks on paper. Then, try the variants out on friends to see if they can easily recognize and pronounce the names.

Nicknames

As you narrow your search, anticipate any nicknames that could arise from both the name on its own as well as the first name and the last name together. It's inevitable that your child will receive several nicknames throughout her life (and some will have nothing to do with her name), so try to think of the ones that could have a negative effect. But don't let this scare you out of using the name you've fallen in love with. Unless they're obvious, most of the drawback names will probably never come up on the playground.

If you like a nickname and not its full name, consider using the nickname as the full name: Abbey instead of Abigail, Kate instead of Katherine, Jen instead of Jennifer. Or, you might consider using the full version of the name anyway to give your child the option of using it in a professional manner for résumés, interviews, and in titles like Dr. Veronica Green instead of Dr. Ronnie Green. Full names are formal and sound more professional. For that reason, people tend to enlist the services of professionals with more sophisticated names. See if you can tell the difference in the following sentence: *After having my taxes done by Charlotte, I played soccer with Charlie.* That's not to say that Charlie wouldn't have prepared your taxes as accurately as Charlotte would, or that Charlotte wouldn't be fun to play soccer with. However, the names create different images in our minds because one is casual and the other is formal.

Full names tend to demand more respect and are more influential, whereas casual nicknames are associated with fun, relaxation, and lightheartedness. When Mom calls Charlie by her full name, it usually means one thing—trouble. And when she calls her by her full first name and her middle name, she quickly learns that Mom means business!

15 Essentials for Finding and Choosing Names

The following are a few suggestions to help make the decision a little easier on you and your entire family.

Say the Names Out Loud

Often we think we like something, but then once we say it out loud, we realize it just isn't what we are looking for. This also works in the opposite way: you think you don't like a name until you say it out loud, and then realize it was exactly what you were looking for. Think of calling loudly for your children on the playground or to come in from playing outside for dinner. If you cringe when doing this, that name probably is not what you were looking for. You need to make sure you say all your children's names together to see if they flow well. They shouldn't be overly similar or drastically dissimilar. Instead, find names that are harmonious without being singsongy.

Avoid Negative Namesakes

When choosing a name, steer clear of names that remind you of people you do not care for or that remind you of an ex-love. These names can only cause you problems in the future. You don't want to forever look at your daughter and think of that one Katherine from grade school who picked on you!

Say All Names Together

Say the name with not only the middle name, but with just the last name. We don't always use our children's middle names, but always use the last name, and if they don't sound right together or come out smoothly together, you need to keep looking.

Test Nicknames

Can your child's name hold up to the playground test? Are there ways that kids can turn the name into something awful that would crush your child's self-esteem and possibly brand her for life? Remember, kids can be cruel, especially siblings. Also make sure that your children won't have the same nicknames. This can happen if the names are too similar or if you use a feminine form of a masculine name for a girl and the masculine name itself for a boy.

Make It Meaningful

Your child's name should be something that makes you feel good. It should reflect qualities that you hope your child will someday possess. Be sure that every child's name is meaningful, not just one. For instance, little Claudia might become resentful if she finds out her name means "one who is lame" while her sister Keisha's name means "the favorite child."

Keep in Mind Spelling and Pronunciations

Names that are difficult to spell and pronounce will be misspelled and mispronounced throughout the child's entire life. Also, keep in mind that using lengthy first names, middle names, and last names all together can be very difficult for a young child to learn to spell and say. An example would be Arabella Margaux Klingele. The poor child would have to learn almost the entire alphabet to spell her name.

Be Creative

Try spelling names of things backward; many unique names can be discovered by doing this. For instance, the name Heaven produces the name Nevaeh. Also play around with dropping letters from established names to create new and unique names that you maybe hadn't thought of. For instance, Mackenzie can become Kenzie, and Jasmine can become Jamine.

Use Maiden Names

A popular way of creating a baby name is by using the mother's maiden name or the maiden name of family members. Mackenzie and Carter are good examples. This is also very popular for middle names as well.

Combine the Parents' Names

Another popular way of coming up with a baby name is by combining parts of the mother's and father's names. Jack and Anna might become Jana, or Grayson and Casey might be Gracie. This is done for both the first and middle names. However, if you do this, make sure you can also create a combined name for another child. Don't play favorites with names; it can affect the self-esteem of and relationship between siblings.

Try Out Different Spellings

You might like a name, but not care for the spelling, thinking it is perhaps too drab or too common. In being creative, anything goes. Stephanie might become Stefani; Lee Ann might become Leighann; Hailey might become Hayleigh. But keep in mind that a child who has an unusual spelling will likely have to correct others over and over during her life.

Explore Genealogy

Another good way to find names is by exploring your family's genealogy. Do a family tree on both the baby's mother's side of the family and the baby's father's side, going back as far as you can. You might need some help from family members with this. Be sure to get the first, middle, and last names of everyone. Then go through these and look for names that stand out to you as something you would like to use. However, when doing this, keep in mind that some people are considered the black sheep of the family. If you settle on a name, be sure to get some background info on this person. You wouldn't want to name your baby something that reminds your mother of the person she most despises. This not only gives you some different names to choose from, but, if you keep it, would be a good gift for your children to have later. Kids love to hear about their ancestors. Again, consider choosing a name from your family tree for each child, not just one.

Ask for Suggestions

Talk to coworkers, neighbors, relatives, and friends. You don't have to use their opinions, but you will receive a ton of suggestions. Also ask them about people who have recently had babies and what those people named their children. This will not only give you name ideas, but will also tell you the names that are being used the most often.

Scour the Media

Consider names from books, television shows, movies, and celebrities. This can be a lot of fun, if you let it.

Consider the Classics

As a general rule of thumb, if your last name is unusual, it's a good idea to choose a more traditional first name. And if you have a common last name, choose a more distinctive first name. Sara Rothberry and Cleora Miller are some examples.

Look to Old-Fashioned Names

These names are making a comeback. They can be good choices because they have the ability to be both distinct and common. Names such as Hazel and Mabel are both easily pronounced and spelled, but are not so common that there would be several in the same classroom.

Have Fun with It!

If you try to have fun and keep the task of choosing a name light, it will go much more smoothly. Making games out of the task is an easy way to take some of the stress off. Here are some game ideas that can be played with just a few people in the privacy of your home, or can be used at a baby shower or gender reveal to get guests to help with the process.

Find a piece of cardboard; it can even be an old cereal box opened up and laid out flat, plain side up. Make a game board similar to Monopoly or Candy Land, using baby names in the squares. You can use different coins or anything you choose for markers. Use a die and take turns rolling it to move around the board. Whoever gets to the end first gets to choose a name from the board to use. Play it four times, choosing four girl names to consider at the end.

Play Scrabble using the rule that you can only make baby names from the letters.

Take a piece of paper, and down one side put the letters of the alphabet, A–Z. Photocopy enough for each guest. Set a time limit and tell everyone to come up with a different or unique name for each letter. At the end, have guests read off the names they have, and any that match should be crossed off. The guest with the most names left wins a prize. The couple gets to keep these pages at the end to give them name ideas to choose from.

Take ten baby names; scramble the letters onto a piece of paper. Photocopy enough for each guest. Set a time limit and see who can come up with the most names using these letters. The couple keeps this at the end to refer to.

Write down the first and last name of the mother and father. Photocopy enough for each guest. Set a time limit and have each guest make names that begin with each letter of their names. Have the guests mark off any that match and see who has the most left at the end. The couple keeps this at the end to give them ideas.

Although this may seem like a long and extremely difficult task, keeping the spotlight on this joyous occasion will help. Try not to put so much pressure on yourself to have that exact and perfect name before the birth. This is not a task that should cause turmoil in the family, but joy.

Remember that naming your child is something that has been entrusted to you, by your baby.

Names with Meaning

A name is more than just the sum of its letters—virtually every moniker is imbued with a particular meaning. Whether it's an attribute, personality trait, season, person, quality, place, or even product, the names you're thinking about have an inherent connection to other concepts. Discovering the meaning behind the names on your list is all part of the fun of naming your little girl. Since names can mean different things in different places and to different people, it's worth putting in some time to learn as much as you can about the name you've chosen, both as a way to prevent negative associations and also as a source of inspiration.

Many parents-to-be cite meaning above all other attributes of a name as their primary inspiration for choosing it. In fact, deciding on a meaning first and then deciding on a name from the pool of contenders is a nice way to choose a firstborn's name, and possibly even other siblings' names down the road. There are two ways to approach this. You can start with an idea you love in a general way—say, for example, peace—and find out which names fit that concept, as Erin, Frieda, and Winifred do. Alternately, you can build from a more personal meaning that reflects your family specifically. If you're both army officers, for example, try Matilda, Louise, or Tyra, all of which mean "great in battle."

Of course, meanings needn't always be hidden or obscure. Virtue names are an excellent example of this idea—names like Faith, Grace, Hope, and Honor certainly do put meaning front and center. There are also more spiritual names, like the classic Mary and Rebecca, or the more unique Genesis and Nevaeh to evoke a specific meaning in your name choice. Wherever you find inspiration, try to choose a name that means something special to you and reflects positive attributes in general.

Do you have any particular attributes (strength, wisdom, courage) that you'd like her name to highlight? List them here and see if you can discover some new options that mean the most to you!

....

....

....

....

....

....

....

....

....

....

....

....

INSPIRATIONAL NAMES

Amity	Genesis	Justice	True
Angel	Grace	Mercy	Verity
Blessing	Harmony	Peace	
Charity	Honor	Serenity	
Dream	Hope	Sincerity	
Faith	Integrity	Trinity	

BIBLICAL NAMES

Abra	Dinah	Mary	Shiloh
Abigail	Eve	Rachel	
Delilah	Leah	Rebecca	

Variations on a Theme

Some groups of names go naturally together, and choosing from within a particular theme is a great way to narrow down the options or pick names for multiples or siblings. Try saint names like Cecilia, Catherine, and Joan, or go more inspirational with Grace and Harmony.

NAMES THAT MEAN "WISE"

Athena	Keyla	Monique	Sennet
Avery	Landra	Rayna	
Dara	Medora	Sage	

NAMES THAT MEAN "LIGHT"

Aileen	Kria	Meira	Ora
Elaine	Liora	Nell	
Jelena	Lucy	Nora	

NAMES THAT MEAN "BLESSING" OR "GIFT" ··················

Adora	Dottie	Joanna	Trixie
Grace	Iva	Mattea	
Darona	Ivana	Thea	

NAMES THAT MEAN "BEAUTIFUL" ··················

Alaina	Belinda	Caiomhe	Memphis
Arabella	Bella	Calista	
Ayanna	Bonnie	Hermosa	

NAMES THAT MEAN "STRONG" ··················

Amalda	Charla	Maude	Sela
Andrea	Chriselda	Megan	Sloane
Audrey	Jerica	Mirit	Tisha
Briana	Karla	Nina	Trudy
Bridget	Keren	Petronelle	Valerie

ROYALTY NAMES ··················

Blessing	Kensington	Princeton	Royalty
Duchess	Kingsley	Queen	
Jewel	Princess	Reign	

SAINT NAMES

Bernadette	Clare	Joan	Teresa
Catherine	Faustina	Margaret	
Cecilia	Felicity	Rose	

NAMES FOR GODDESSES

Aphrodite	Demeter	Hestia	Selene
Artemis	Eirene	Nike	
Athena	Hera	Persephone	

Unique Inspiration

There are people who like popular names, and there are people who don't. While one set of parents-to-be might choose the name Ava because it consistently ranks among the top ten girls' names, there are others who'd stay away from Ava for precisely that reason. For the latter group, there are plenty of other places to look for a unique name for your future daughter.

From specific sounds to unique categories, fantastic naming inspiration is everywhere! Look through some of your favorite books and movies—are there any characters or actors with unique names? What about a particular region—are you looking for something with a southern flair, or maybe some northeastern posh? What about playing around with spelling, finding a nickname that you love and using it as your girl's first name, or using some fantastic variants of popular favorites (Ellspeth for Elizabeth, Avalyn for Ava)? The possibilities are endless.

Blending Favorites

Maybe you've narrowed it down to two choices and can't decide, or perhaps you simply want your little one's name to reflect both her parents: Taylor and Lia became Talia, Chris and Ellen become Chriselle, Will and Olivia become Willa. It's a super-original way to make sure your little girl's name has the most meaning!

Here are some more places to look for unique names you may (or may not) find on any top 100 list:

SOUTHERN NAMES

Adeline	Dallas	June	Virginia
Caroline	Dixie	Loretta	
Daisy	Ella-Mae	Presley	

PREPPY NAMES

Ainsley	Cornelia	Lennox	Sloane
Blair	Darcy	Margaux	Sterling
Bronwyn	Ellison	Palmer	Teague
Carlisle	Finley	Parker	Tilly
Collins	Leighton	Poppy	Tinsley

CONSTELLATIONS

Agitta	Aquila	Lyra	Vela
Andromeda	Carina	Norma	
Antila	Hydra	Ursa	

NICKNAMES AS NAMES

Addie	Coco	Kat	Quinn
Alli	Edie	Mac	Remy
Bea	Ellie	Maggie	Sam
Bella	Gale	Millie	Tori
Betsy	Gigi	Olive	Winnie

COLORS

Azura	Iris	Ruby	Violet
Ebony	Mauve	Russet	
Emerald	Olive	Scarlet	

SHAKESPEAREAN NAMES

Adriana	Cordelia	Olivia	Rosalind
Bianca	Helena	Ophelia	
Celia	Juliet	Portia	

NATURE NAMES

Aspen	Daisy	Ivy	Rose
Autumn	Delta	Magnolia	Sierra
Birdie	Hazel	Oaklynn	Wilder
Briar	Hunter	Rain	Willow
Calla	Iris	River	Wren

GRANDMA NAMES

Agnes	Evelyn	Mabel	Virginia
Dorothy	Florence	Margaret	
Elsie	Irene	Mildred	

What are some of your favorite books? Are there any character names that you love?

LITERARY HEROINES

Ada	Cosette	Harper	Melba
Anais	Daisy	Hermione	Penelope
Anna	Eliza	Hester	Scarlett
Brett	Elizabeth	Holly	Scout
Clarissa	Estella	Maya	Sula

CHILDREN'S LIT NAMES

Alice	Eloise	Lucy	Nancy
Amelia	Ginny	Madeline	Pippi
Arrietty	Harriet	Mary Anne	Ramona
Beatrice	Jo	Matilda	Sophie
Charlotte	Laura	Meg	Susan

FANDOM NAMES

Arwen	Ginny	Luna	Uhura
Arya	Khaleesi	Rey	
Diana	Leia	Sansa	

CLASSIC NAMES

Alexandra	Jane	Patricia	Vivian
Charlotte	Katherine	Rebecca	
Ellen	Margaret	Susannah	

FLAVORFUL NAMES

Brie	Honey	Rosemary	Thyme
Clementine	Pepper	Saffron	
Ginger	Poppy	Sage	

NAMES ON THE RISE

Amora	Kehlani	Melania	Yara
Ensley	Lyanna	Paisleigh	
Emberly	Maren	Selene	

NAMES THAT END IN -LEE

Bailee	Haylee	Novalee	Zaylee
Brynlee	Kaylee	Paislee	
Charlee	Kynlee	Rylee	

········ Top Alternatives to the Top 10 ········

If you like an extremely popular name but wish it were more unique, here are some fresh alternatives you may find appealing.

Instead of Emma, try...

Amelie	Jemma	Romily
Emeline	Milly	

Instead of Olivia, try...

Alivia   Lydia   Olive

Lilah   Odelia

Instead of Ava, try...

Ada   Avelyn   Aviva

Avanna   Avery

Instead of Isabella, try...

Anabell   Isild   Sabelle

Gabriella   Isolde

Instead of Sophia, try...

Lucia   Seraphina   Sylvia

Sadie   Sofi

Instead of Mia, try...

Amia   Mina   Tia

Esme   Mya

Instead of Charlotte, try...

Caroline   Charlise   Scarlett

Charlene   Lottie

Instead of Amelia, try...

Amelie	Emmeline	Melia
Ania	Emmylou	

Instead of Evelyn, try...

Adelyn	Evangeline	Vivienne
Aveline	Lenora	

Instead of Abigail, try...

Abilene	Audrey	Libby
Abra	Greta	

Anything that sparked your interest? What are some of your favorite trendy names? List them here.

....

....

....

....

....

....

....

....

....

Famous Influence

C ertain names evoke certain feelings in people, which is often why we turn to some of our favorite, and most famous, friends for naming inspiration. Whether it be your favorite sports star, a powerful female scientist, an exemplary author, or the celebrity or singer you look up to the most, famous names are often a great place to start when you're looking to name your future daughter.

However, one thing to keep in mind: whether fictional or not, certain names are forever embedded in our psyche as having very specific character traits or legacies. You'll need to remember these associations when creating the name that your child will live with for the rest of her life. Like it or not, Oprah, Madonna, Aretha, Hillary, Beyoncé, and Rosa will always bring to mind the personalities they're most often associated with. If you adore the legacy these names have left behind, then forge ahead!

Here are some famous female powerhouses to browse through:

ACTIVISTS

Alice	Bell	Gloria	Rosa
Angela	Eleanor	Harriet	
Audre	Emma	Malala	

COUNTRY SINGERS

Carrie	June	Loretta	Shania
Dolly	Kacey	Maren	
Faith	LeAnn	Miranda	

CLASSIC MOVIE STARS

Audrey	Elizabeth	Judy	Marlene
Ava	Gene	Katherine	Myrna
Bette	Greta	Loren	Natalie
Brigitte	Ingrid	Lucille	Rita
Claudette	Joan	Marilyn	Vivien

POP STAR NAMES

Aretha	Christina	Taylor
Ariana	Madonna	Whitney
Beyoncé	Mariah	
Camila	Selena	

FASHION DESIGNERS

Betsey	Donatella	Stella	Vivienne
Carolina	Donna	Tory	
Coco	Kate	Vera	

PRESIDENTIAL NAMES

Carter	James	McKinley	Taylor
Hayes	Kennedy	Monroe	
Jackson	Madison	Reagan	

Art Attack

Scour your favorite movies, books, and music for ideas. Jazz fans may want to choose Ella or Billie; art lovers, Frida or Joan; cinema connoisseurs, Sofia or Kathryn.

ARTISTS

Adrian	Georgia	Louise
Agnes	Helen	Yayoi
Élisabeth	Mary	
Frida	Minnie	

COMEDIANS

Amy	Julia	Sarah	Whoopi
Betty	Kristen	Tina	
Ellen	Lucille	Wanda	

POETS

Anne	Gertrude	Mary	Sylvia
Audre	Gwendolyn	Maya	
Emily	Lucille	Rupi	

SPORTS LEGENDS

Billie	Jackie	Maria	Simone
Bonnie	Lindsey	Mia	
Danica	Lisa	Serena	

SCIENTISTS

Ada	Grace	Lise	Stephanie
Caroline	Hedy	Marie	
Emilie	Irène	Rosalind	

CELEBRITY NAMES

Brie	Julia	Octavia	Saoirse
Constance	Margot	Reese	
Gal	Meryl	Salma	

What are some of your favorite famous inspira-tions? Any names you may want to adopt for your own little one?

....

....

....

....

....

....

....

....

....

....

....

....

....

....

....

....

....

....

....

....

....

Celebrity Baby Names A–Z

Our society is fascinated with the names celebrities choose for their children. Any new celebrity birth instantly makes headlines. So, whether you're looking for inspiration or you're just curious, here's an alphabetical listing of baby names and the celebrities who chose them.

Agnes Charles

Elisabeth Shue and Davis Guggenheim

Alabama Gypsy Rose

Drea de Matteo and Shooter Jennings

Amada Lee

Eva Mendes and Ryan Gosling

Apple Blythe Alison

Gwyneth Paltrow and Chris Martin

Aquinnah Kathleen

Tracy Pollan and Michael J. Fox

Ashby Grace

Nancy O'Dell and Keith Zubchevich

Aviana Olea

Amy Adams and Darren Le Gallo

Avri Roel

Susan Downey and Robert Downey Jr.

Bandit Lee

Lyn-Z Way and Gerard Way

Birdie Leigh

Busy Philipps and Marc Silverstein

Blue Ivy

Beyoncé and Jay-Z

Briar Rose

Rachel Bilson and Hayden Christensen

Calico

Sheryl Cooper and Alice Cooper

Carys Zeta

Catherine Zeta-Jones and Michael Douglas

Sam Alexis

Elin Nordegren and Tiger Woods

Coco Riley

Courteney Cox and David Arquette

D'Lila Star

Kim Porter and Sean Combs

Daisy Josephine

Olivia Wilde and Jason Sudeikis

Delta Bell

Kristen Bell and Dax Shepard

Destry Allyn

Kate Capshaw and Steven Spielberg

Dexter

Diane Keaton

Dixie Pearl

Lily Aldridge and Caleb Followill

Dream Renée

Blac Chyna and Rob Kardashian

Dusty Rose

Behati Prinsloo and Adam Levine

Emerson Rose

Teri Hatcher and Jon Tenney

Emme Maribel

Jennifer Lopez and Marc Anthony

Etta Jones

Siri Pinter and Carson Daly

Eve Sunny Day

Ali Hewson and Bono

Evelyn Penn

Emma Heming-Willis and Bruce Willis

Fifi Trixibelle

Paula Yates and Bob Geldof

Finley Aaron Love

Lisa Marie Presley and Michael Lockwood

Frances Cole

Nancy Juvonen and Jimmy Fallon

Francesca Nora

Amanda Anka and Jason Bateman

Galen Grier

Victoria Duffy and Dennis Hopper

Gemma Rose

Kristin Davis

Georgia Tatum

Jill Goodacre and Harry Connick Jr.

Gia Zavala

Luciana Barroso and Matt Damon

Gianna Maria-Onore

Vanessa Laine Bryant and Kobe Bryant

Gloria Ray

Maggie Gyllenhaal and Peter Sarsgaard

Harlow Winter Kate

Nicole Richie and Joel Madden

Harper Seven

Victoria Beckham and David Beckham

Hattie Margaret

Tori Spelling and Dean McDermott

Haven Garner

Jessica Alba and Cash Warren

Hazel

Emily Blunt and John Krasinski

Honor Marie

Jessica Alba and Cash Warren

Inez

Blake Lively and Ryan Reynolds

Iris Mary

Hannah Bagshawe and Eddie Redmayne

Isadora

Björk and Matthew Barney

Isla

Paula Radcliffe and Gary Lough

Italia Anita Maria

Simone Johnson and LL Cool J

Jaz Elle

Steffi Graf and Andre Agassi

Jennifer Katharine

Melinda Gates and Bill Gates

Jessie James

Kim Porter and Sean Combs

Jillian Kristin

Vanessa Williams and Ramon Hervey

Johnnie Rose

Melissa Etheridge and Tammy Lynn Michaels

Jolie Rae

Jana Kramer and Michael Caussin

Justice

Victoria Granucci and John Mellencamp

Kadence Clover

Lhotse Merriam and Tony Hawk

Kaya Evdokia

Hayden Panettiere and Wladimir Klitschko

Kimber Lynn

Roxanne Tunis and Clint Eastwood

Liberty Irene

Jean Kasem and Casey Kasem

Lila Grace

Kate Moss and Jefferson Hack

Liv Helen

Julianne Moore and Bart Freundlich

Lola Simone

Malaak Compton-Rock and Chris Rock

Lou Sulola

Heidi Klum and Seal

Luca Bella

Jennie Garth and Peter Facinelli

Luna Simone

Chrissy Teigen and John Legend

Maddie Briann

Jamie Lynn Spears and Casey Aldridge

Maggie Rose

Tracey McShane and Jon Stewart

Marlowe Ottoline Layng

Sienna Miller and Tom Sturridge

Matilda Rose

Michelle Williams and Heath Ledger

Memphis Eve

Ali Hewson and Bono

Nahla Ariela

Halle Berry and Gabriel Aubry

Natalia Diamante

Vanessa Laine Bryant and Kobe Bryant

Nell

Helena Bonham Carter and Tim Burton

Nia

Tomeeka Robyn Bracy and Stevie Wonder

North

Kim Kardashian and Kanye West

Odette

Sunrise Coigney and Mark Ruffalo

Olive

Isla Fisher and Sacha Baron Cohen

Ophelia Saint

Jordyn Blum and Dave Grohl

Penelope Scotland

Kourtney Kardashian and Scott Disick

Petal Blossom Rainbow

Jools Oliver and Jamie Oliver

Piper Maru

Gillian Anderson and Clyde Klotz

Poet Sienna Rose

Soleil Moon Frye and Jason Goldberg

Poppy Honey Rosie

Jools Oliver and Jamie Oliver

Puma Sabti

Erykah Badu and Tracy Curry

Reign Beau

Deborah Reed and Ving Rhames

River Rose

Kelly Clarkson and Brandon Blackstock

Romy

Sofia Coppola and Thomas Mars

Rosalind Arusha Arkadina Altalune Florence

Uma Thurman and Arpad Busson

Rose Dorothy

Scarlett Johansson and Romain Dauriac

Ruby Sweetheart

Jennifer Meyer and Tobey Maguire

Sadie Madison

Jackie Sandler and Adam Sandler

Sam Alexis

Elin Nordegren and Tiger Woods

Savannah

Marcia Cross and Tom Mahoney

Scarlet Rose

Jennifer Flavin and Sylvester Stallone

Seraphina Rose Elizabeth

Jennifer Garner and Ben Affleck

Shiloh Nouvel

Angelina Jolie and Brad Pitt

Sienna May

Ellen Pompeo and Chris Ivery

Sistine Rose

Jennifer Flavin and Sylvester Stallone

Stella Luna

Ellen Pompeo and Chris Ivery

Stormi Webster

Kylie Jenner and Travis Scott

Sunday Rose

Nicole Kidman and Keith Urban

Sunny Madeline

Jackie Sandler and Adam Sandler

Suri

Katie Holmes and Tom Cruise

Tabitha Hodge

Sarah Jessica Parker and Matthew Broderick

Tallulah Belle

Demi Moore and Bruce Willis

True

Khloé Kardashian and Tristan Thompson

Valentina Paloma

Salma Hayek and François-Henri Pinault

Vera Audrey

Emilie de Ravin and Eric Bilitch

Victoria

Yvette Prieto Jordan and Michael Jordan

Vida

Camila Alves and Matthew McConaughey

Violet

Emily Blunt and John Krasinski

Vivian Lake

Gisele Bündchen and Tom Brady

Willa

Mimi O'Donnell and Philip Seymour Hoffman

Wyatt Isabelle

Mila Kunis and Ashton Kutcher

Wynter Merin

Tawny Kitaen and Chuck Finley

Ysabel

Yvette Prieto Jordan and Michael Jordan

Zahara Marley

Angelina Jolie and Brad Pitt

Zoe Grace

Kimberly Quaid and Dennis Quaid

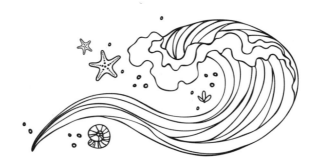

Unisex Favorites

Unisex names have been around for ages, but they are just now pushing their way to the forefront of popularity. This could be due to the fact that there are more parents who want to strip their children of gender restraints. For instance, when the résumé of Jordan Smith crosses the HR director's desk, there will be no way for him or her to tell whether Jordan is a man or woman, and therefore all gender bias has been erased. Jordan will have to secure that interview on merit alone. On the other hand, some parents choose unisex names because of the associations they carry. For instance, parents may want their daughter's name to embody strength and power; after all, she's going to be a beauty already, so why would she need a feminine name to reiterate that? Choosing a more masculine name may accomplish this.

Some parents want to give their children names that are a bit unusual, those that will set their children apart in the sea of Emmas and Marys. Unisex names break away from traditional feminine names, adding to the pot a variety of choices that will make the classroom roster a bit more colorful. There is also a wide variety of meanings to choose from. Whether you are looking for a name from nature, a place name, a name meaning "strength," a name meaning "beauty," or a name meaning "benevolence," you can find it in the list of unisex names available today.

Or maybe you'd prefer to bring a name to the unisex list. If you are expecting a daughter, you might want to browse boys' names and see if there is one that sounds as though it has an ounce of femininity to it. Names that end in an *ie*, *ee*, or *ey* typically have a feminine sound to them. Maybe the feminine sound isn't at all important, and you'd rather name your daughter Robert. The choice is entirely yours; there are no rules when it comes to baby naming. However, you will likely want to take into consideration the consequences of the name you choose.

A unisex name is one that can be used for either gender. Lots of names are popular for both boys and girls, but they're generally more popular for one gender than the other. Historically, most unisex names began as boys' names but for one reason or another began to appeal to parents of girls. Once it becomes common for girls to take on these names, they become unisex, though sometimes, the pattern works in reverse. Names such as Lindsay and

Florence are true unisex names, as they have their roots in masculinity, but they have been so predominantly used for girls that they are considered to be part of the girls' names list and are no longer often seen as an option for boys. The following is a list of the top unisex names—names that appear in both the boys' and girls' top 1,000 names as compiled by the Social Security Administration. We've broken these up by how predominately they are used by girls versus boys.

NEARLY EQUAL

Charlie	Landry	River	Skyler
Justice	Oakley	Rowan	

MORE POPULAR FOR GIRLS

Alexis	Finley	London	Reese
Ariel	Harley	Lyric	Riley
Avery	Harper	Marley	Sage
Dakota	Jamie	Morgan	Skylar
Eden	Jessie	Nova	Sutton
Emerson	Kendall	Payton	Tatum
Emery	Leighton	Peyton	Taylor
Emory	Lennon	Quinn	

OTHER OPTIONS

Amari	Dallas	Jordan	Remy
Angel	Dylan	Kai	Rory
Ari	Elliot	Micah	Royal
Blake	Ellis	Lennox	Ryan
Cameron	Hayden	Logan	Rylan
Carter	Hunter	Parker	Sawyer
Casey	Jayden	Phoenix	Zion

Spelling Matters!

If you're going to choose…

Cameron/Camryn/Kamryn: Camryn and Kamryn are the more popular choices for girls, Cameron for boys

Skylar/Skyler: Skylar is more popular for girls, while Skyler wins for boys

Jordan/Jordyn: Jordyn is more popular for girls, Jordan for boys

UNDER THE RADAR

Arlo	Frankie	Jules	Wyatt
Brett	Gray	Monroe	
Delta	James	Stevie	

What are some boy names you love? Did you just find the perfect gender-neutral option for your little girl?

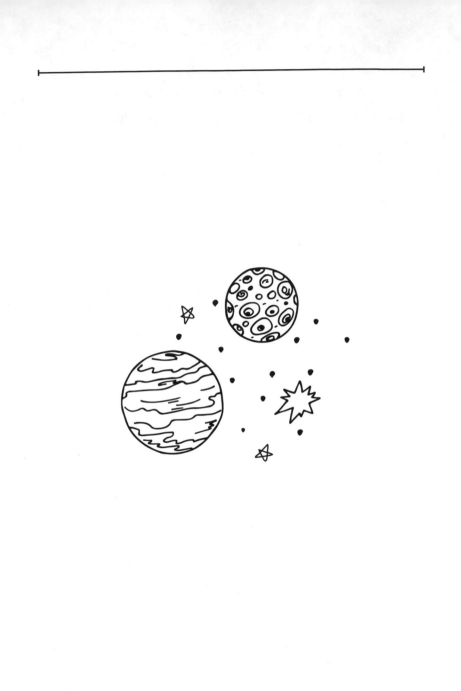

Around the World

In this era of globalization, baby-name trends are not immune to worldwide influence. While many parents choose to honor their roots by selecting a name from their own ethnic background, it appears that having a familial connection to an ethnicity is not a prerequisite for choosing a name from that ethnicity. This is actually not a brand-new trend; it has happened before that one ethnicity's names take on a mainstream popularity for a period of time. For instance, names of Hispanic origin became popular in the sixties, leading to the rise in popularity of names like Juanita among non-Hispanics. However, never before has the average parent had access to such a wide variety of names. Here are just a few places you can look when naming your new little one.

Celtic Names

Americans specifically have long held a fascination with Celtic culture. Recently, this interest has grown in magnitude and strength, helped along by the rising popularity of Celtic literature, music, and dance, and the fact that so many Americans trace their roots back to the Celtic strongholds of Wales, England, Ireland, and Scotland. Many of these names have grown in popularity so much that they have lost the slightly odd, new feeling many names from other countries have. Many new Celtic names have been increasingly breaking into the ranks of common American baby names.

From Ireland, some of the more popular girls' names are Aisling, Briana, Ciara, Caoimhe, Fiona, Moira, Niamh, Shannon, and Siobhan.

Scottish girls' names include Amie, Abbie, Isla, Seonaid, Tam, Morag, Lorna, Aileen, and Edme.

Wales is also a prominent source for Celtic names today. Some increasingly popular Welsh names for girls are Meredith, Guinevere, Rhonwen, Rhiannon, Catrin, Bryn, Freya, Phoebe, and Carys.

Other Celtic peoples, such as the Bretons and Cornish, also contribute to the Celtic naming trend but not yet on the scale that the others do. Here's a look at some of our Celtic favorites.

POPULAR NAMES IN IRELAND

Aoife	Ellie	Roisin	Sophia
Caoimhe	Grace	Sadie	
Chloe	Kate	Saoirse	

POPULAR NAMES IN SCOTLAND

Anna	Greer	Imogen	Skye
Aria	Eilidh	Kirstine	
Ayla	Ellie	Orla	

POPULAR NAMES IN WALES

Ariana	Efa	Elin	Nansi
Bonnie	Eleanor	Gwen	
Darcey	Eleri	Madison	

British Names

One can argue that Britain and the United States draw from a nearly similar name pool. However, certain names are used in each country that are rarely used in the other. With the success of many British authors, notably J. K. Rowling (*Harry Potter*) and Helen Fielding (*Bridget Jones*), and British films and television programs in the United States, some of these uniquely British names have been working their way into American popular consciousness and thus into baby-naming trends as well. This is true particularly for girls, with names like Poppy, Gemma, Nicola, Maisie, Pippa, and Tamzin appearing in the United States.

POPULAR NAMES IN ENGLAND ··

Darcy	Florence	Lola	Poppy
Eleanor	Imogen	Millie	
Fatima	Lily	Olivia	

African Names

Obviously, Africa is a continent of many nations and peoples, and accordingly a source of great variety of names and naming customs. In recent times, many Americans of African descent have looked to Africa for names that represent their history and culture and their pride therein. However, African names have also been shown to appeal to a broader spectrum of the public. There is a wide variety of sources for traditional African names, including information about the origin and meanings. Since there are so many distinct cultures and peoples in Africa, we will just list a few of the more well-known names in America for girls: Baina, Kali, Malia, Radhi, and Zaina.

POPULAR NAMES IN NIGERIA

Adaeze	Daraja	Lewa	Sade
Amadi	Eya	Omorosa	
Aretta	Ife	Rayowa	

POPULAR NAMES IN SOUTH AFRICA

Amahle	Enzokuhle	Melokuhle	Thandolwethu
Amogelang	Lethabo	Omphile	
Blessing	Lutando	Precious	

What is your own heritage? Are there any names from that country or culture that have always stuck out to you?

....

....

....

....

....

....

....

....

....

....

Popular Names Around the World

Let's take a look at some other popular favorites from across the globe.

POPULAR NAMES IN AUSTRALIA

Amelia	Indi	Matilda	Zara
Evie	Isla	Thea	
Freya	Layla	Willow	

POPULAR NAMES IN BRAZIL

Antonia	Elena	Isadora	Valentina
Beatriz	Eloa	Pietra	
Catarina	Feliciana	Raissa	

POPULAR NAMES IN CANADA

Abigail	Isabella	Mia	Zoey
Ava	Madison	Nora	
Emma	Maya	Riley	

POPULAR NAMES IN FRANCE

Camille	Juliette	Manon	Océane
Chloé	Lina	Marie	
Jade	Louise	Marine	

POPULAR NAMES IN GERMANY

Alina	Helena	Luisa	Pia
Frieda	Lina	Marie	
Greta	Lotta	Marlene	

POPULAR NAMES IN ISRAEL

Adele	Maya	Shira	Yael
Avigail	Noa	Talia	
Esther	Sarah	Tamar	

POPULAR NAMES IN ITALY

Alessia	Chiara	Martina	Sofia
Aurora	Giulia	Nicole	
Beatrice	Greta	Sara	

POPULAR NAMES IN JAPAN

Akari	Kaede	Mio	Yui
An	Kokoha	Riko	
Himari	Mei	Sakura	

POPULAR NAMES IN NEW ZEALAND

Amelia	Charlotte	Isla	Sophia
Ayla	Emily	Maisie	
Bella	Harper	Mila	

POPULAR NAMES IN NORWAY

Alma	Emilie	Norah	Sofie
Amalie	Ingrid	Sara	
Aurora	Maja	Selma	

POPULAR NAMES IN SPAIN

Adriana	Daniela	Lucia	Valeria
Alba	Emma	Maria	
Carla	Laura	Paula	

POPULAR NAMES IN SWEDEN

Agnes	Ebba	Nellie	Wilma
Alice	Elsa	Signe	
Astrid	Julia	Vera	

POPULAR NAMES IN TURKEY

Azra	Ecrin	Hiranur	Zeynep
Defne	Elif	Miray	
Ebrar	Hira	Zehra	

Classic Options

Since the American people are composed of people from many different countries, we can expect a wide variety of names to appear on the landscape, many of which will have broad appeal. Classic names from countries like France (Pascale and Amelie for girls), Germany, and Italy have also increased in popularity. Middle Eastern, Indian, Chinese, Japanese, and other countries and cultures are contributing names on an ever-increasing basis due to the "shrinking globe." Hispanic names, some of which are already quite common, are also increasing in frequency of use. Russian names such as Natasha, Sasha, Ludmila, and Nadia are being used. The names Misha and Nikita are being given as names for female children, even though in Russian they are traditionally male names (Misha being a diminutive for Mikhail).

For parents who are looking into ethnic names, there are numerous websites and books that cover each country or region and give meanings and origins of the names as well. It is particularly important for parents who have little or no background with a certain country or group to look into the meanings and associations with certain names.

AFRICAN NAMES

Asha	Imani	Nailah	Zoya
Bunme	Lulu	Sabra	
Dalia	Malika	Tanesha	

AFRICAN AMERICAN NAMES

Aaliyah	Jayla	Kiara	Nia
Celie	Jordan	Makayla	Raisha
Cherise	Kalinda	Maya	Toni
Imani	Keisha	Nakari	Trinity
Jada	Kenya	Nevaeh	Zora

ARABIC NAMES

Amalia	Hayat	Leila	Zara
Amira	Joelle	Mila	
Farah	Katya	Nadia	

ASIAN NAMES

Akako	Chaitali	Sato	Yori
Aki	Kai	Vanita	
Cam	Rumi	Vanna	

DUTCH NAMES

Annelies	Grete	Maaike	Tess
Beatrix	Hanneke	Maud	
Fay	Lotte	Sanne	

FRENCH NAMES

Adelaide	Benoite	Camille	Estelle
Apolline	Bernadette	Delphine	Fleur

Francine	Juliette	Martine	Simone
Hélène	Margaux	Odette	Violette
Héloïse	Madeleine	Pauline	Yvette

GERMAN NAMES

Bianca	Gretchen	Lenore	Ulla
Clarissa	Heidi	Liesel	
Elsa	Henrietta	Maude	

GREEK NAMES

Ariadne	Hermione	Lyra	Sofi
Calista	Kalliope	Penelope	
Daphne	Leda	Petra	

IRISH NAMES

Aileen	Catriona	Isolde	Siobhán
Aoife	Deirdre	Máire	
Brianna	Eileen	Rhionnan	

ITALIAN NAMES

Alessandra	Francesca	Ottavia	Teresa
Cara	Gia	Serafina	
Elizabetta	Isabella	Simone	

POLISH NAMES

Beatris	Dorota	Lila	Poila
Brygid	Elzbieta	Margita	
Celestyn	Krysta	Renata	

ROMAN NAMES

Antonia	Claudia	Julia	Minerva
Augusta	Flavia	Lucretia	
Clara	Flora	Maxima	

SCOTTISH NAMES

Alba	Cairstine	Innis	Morag
Annis	Elspeth	Iona	
Bonnie	Fiona	Maggie	

SPANISH NAMES

Abril	Gabriela	Magdalena	Vanessa
Alma	Isidora	Natalia	
Constanza	Juana	Paulina	

WELSH NAMES

Arwen	Gwendolyn	Meredith	Wynny
Brynna	Isolde	Morgan	
Carys	Mair	Reese	

Are there any names from around the world that you find striking? Make a list of some of your favorites and where they are from. Is there any country that you're particularly drawn to?

··

··

··

··

··

··

··

··

··

··

··

··

Uniquely American

Americans are a creative people, not bound by tradition and rules. These qualities are expressed in naming as well. Early Americans happily used adjectives describing desired qualities for their children, including Patience, Temperance, Makepeace, and Prudence. Many of these names are making a comeback, along with Hope, Faith, Joy, and Peace. Many popular American names come from American Indian names, words, and tribes (Cheyenne, Dakota, Cherokee). However, parents seeking to name their children one of these names should do their research. There is a lot of folklore surrounding names that is inaccurate, and some names may have special status for American Indians, where naming a child with that name may be disrespectful.

NATIVE AMERICAN TRIBAL NAMES

Apache	Comanche	Seminole	Shoshone
Cherokee	Dakota	Seneca	
Cheyenne	Navajo	Shawnee	

PATRIOTIC NAMES

Abigail	Julia	Starlyn
America	Justice	Starr
Betsy	Liberty	
Freeda	Spirit	

Global Village

It may seem an unlikely approach, but maps, globes, and even road atlases are an amazing source of onomatological wealth. Look to street names, towns, rivers, mountains, and far-off places to yield a rich variety of meanings and sounds. If it's a place you happen to know and love, all the better.

Place Names

Maps have long provided inspiration in the naming of children, whether because the locale had a particular significance to the parents, or just because they liked the way it sounded. Many children share their names with cities, states, countries, and regions.

Celebrities appear to be spearheading the revival of this trend: Madonna named her daughter Lourdes, David Beckham named his son Brooklyn, and then there is Paris Hilton. Names like China and India have been around for a while. Some state names have become quite common, like Virginia, Georgia, and Carolina. Other states are now starting to appear on birth certificates, like Dakota, Indiana, and Montana. Cities are also inspiring parents: Savannah, Austin, Houston, Atlanta, and Phoenix. Even ancient lands and cities, such as Troy and Atlantis, are popular names. Country names often used include Israel,

Cuba, Kenya, and Jordan. Many of these names are considered unisex; some are primarily one or the other depending on whether the sound of the name is more feminine or masculine to the parents.

PLACE NAMES

Adelaide	Charlotte	Kaya	Paris
Aspen	Cheyenne	Kerry	Phoenix
Aurora	Florence	London	Savannah
Brooklyn	Georgia	Lourraine	Sierra
Catalina	Helena	Madeira	Victoria

Top Names Throughout History

Names, like fashion, go in and out of vogue. Each time period seems to have a certain naming style that defines it. Currently, the Courtneys, Chelseas, and Brittanys of the 1990s have been replaced with Emilys, Isabellas, and Mias. So what exactly are the hottest names from the past? Here's a look at the top names from each decade (and some new rising favorites):

MOST POPULAR OF THE 1940S

Barbara	Judith	Nancy	Shirley
Betty	Linda	Patricia	
Carol	Mary	Sandra	

MOST POPULAR OF THE 1950S

Barbara	Kathleen	Nancy	Susan
Carol	Linda	Patricia	
Deborah	Mary	Sandra	

MOST POPULAR OF THE 1960S ·······················

Cynthia	Donna	Lisa	Susan
Deborah	Karen	Mary	
Debra	Linda	Patricia	

MOST POPULAR OF THE 1970S ·······················

Amy	Kimberly	Melissa	Tracy
Angela	Lisa	Michelle	
Jennifer	Mary	Tammy	

MOST POPULAR OF THE 1980S ·······················

Amanda	Heather	Melissa	Sarah
Amy	Jennifer	Michelle	
Elizabeth	Jessica	Nicole	

MOST POPULAR OF THE 1990S ·······················

Amanda	Elizabeth	Lauren	Stephanie
Ashley	Jennifer	Samantha	
Brittany	Jessica	Sarah	

MOST POPULAR OF 2000S ·······················

Alexis	Emily	Madison	Taylor
Ashley	Hannah	Samantha	
Elizabeth	Jessica	Sarah	

MOST POPULAR OF 2010 ···

Abigail	Emily	Madison	Sophia
Ava	Emma	Mia	
Chloe	Isabella	Olivia	

MOST POPULAR NAMES OF 2015 ·································

Abigail	Emily	Isabella	Sophia
Ava	Emma	Mia	
Charlotte	Harper	Olivia	

MOST POPULAR NAMES EXPECTED IN 2020 ··············

Ava	Emma	Isabella	Sophia
Avery	Evelyn	Mia	
Charlotte	Harper	Olivia	

NAMES ON THE RISE ···

Alora	India	Oaklyn	Spencer
Aminah	Legacy	Octavia	Xiomara
Amora	Luella	Paisleigh	
Emerald	Marlowe	Saanvi	
Everlee	Melania	Selene	
Dream	Mylah	Sonia	

NAMES UNDER THE RADAR ·······································

Alessia	Calliope	Everleigh	Paloma
Alma	Davina	Frankie	Reina
Amora	Demi	Kynlee	Stevie
Ari	Ellis	Mabel	Tinsley
Belle	Emmie	Maren	Zaria

Names from A to Z

~⌒~

Do you want your future daughter's name to start with the same letter as yours? Or maybe you want your little girl's name to start with the most (or least) popular letter of the alphabet? You may find it surprising, but recently only nine of the top 1,000 girl baby names start with an O: Oaklee, Oakley, Oaklyn, Oaklynn, Octavia, Olive, Olivia, Opal, and Ophelia. At the same time, you probably won't find it as surprising that the most popular letter that girls' names start with is A (169 of the top 1,000), with M as a close second with 103 names. Take a look at some other names for each letter:

A NAMES

Abigail	Amelia	Audrina	Azalea
Adelyn	Amira	Ava	
Alena	Anya	Avery	

What does your name start with? Your partner's? List some options for each letter below.

....

....

....

....

....

....

....

....

....

....

....

....

....

....

....

....

....

....

....

....

....

....

B NAMES

Belen	Bonnie	Briar	Brynn
Blaire	Brenna	Bristol	
Blake	Brianna	Brooke	

C NAMES

Carolina	Cecilia	Claire	Cynthia
Casey	Celeste	Collins	
Catalina	Charlie	Cora	

D NAMES

Dahlia	Danica	Demi	Dylan
Daisy	Daphne	Diana	
Dakota	Delilah	Dora	

E NAMES

Eden	Ellis	Emory	Evie
Elaina	Eloise	Esperanza	
Elise	Emmalyn	Everlee	

F NAMES

Faith	Felicity	Frances	Frida
Fatima	Finley	Francesca	
Faye	Fiona	Freya	

G NAMES

Gabriella	Georgia	Gloria	Gwen
Genesis	Giovanna	Grace	
Genevieve	Giselle	Guadalupe	

H NAMES

Hadley	Harlow	Hattie	Hope
Hailey	Harmony	Helen	
Hannah	Harper	Holly	

I NAMES

Imani	Irene	Itzayana	Ivy
India	Iris	Itzel	
Ingrid	Isabelle	Ivory	

J NAMES

Jana	Jennifer	Jolie	Juniper
Jayla	Jilian	Josephine	
Jazlyn	Joanna	Juliana	

K NAMES

Kaia	Kathleen	Kimberly	Kylie
Kaitlyn	Kaylin	Kira	
Karsyn	Khloe	Kori	

L NAMES

Laurel	Leighton	Lola	Lyric
Lauren	Lennox	Louisa	
Legacy	Lilian	Luna	

M NAMES

Mabel	Marina	Melody	Morgan
Madeline	McKinley	Mila	
Maia	Melina	Molly	

N NAMES

Nancy	Nevaeh	Noelle	Nyla
Natalie	Nia	Nora	
Natasha	Nicole	Nova	

O NAMES

Oaklee	Odessa	Olivia	Orion
Oaklynn	Olie	Opal	
Océane	Olive	Ophelia	

P NAMES

Paisley	Parker	Perla	Piper
Paloma	Penelope	Peyton	
Paris	Penny	Phoenix	

Q NAMES

Qeleigh	Queenie	Quincie	Quirien
Quartney	Quilla	Quinlan	
Queen	Quinby	Quinn	

R NAMES

Raelyn	Remington	Riley	Rowan
Ramona	Renata	Rory	
Reese	Rhea	Rosemary	

S NAMES

Sabrina	Savannah	Skylar	Sutton
Salma	Serena	Sophia	
Sarai	Sierra	Sunny	

T NAMES

Talia	Tenley	Tiffany	Trinity
Tatum	Tessa	Tinley	
Taylor	Thalia	Tori	

U NAMES

Udele	Ulyana	Unique	Ursula
Ulla	Uma	Uri	
Ululani	Una	Ursa	

V NAMES

Vada	Vera	Vienna	Vivian
Valeria	Veronica	Violet	
Vanessa	Victoria	Virginia	

W NAMES

Waverly	Wilder	Winnie	Wren
Wells	Willa	Winona	
Whitney	Willow	Winter	

X NAMES

Xabrina	Xenia	Ximena	Xyleena
Xavier	Xerena	Xio	
Xena	Xia	Xiomara	

Y NAMES

Yana	Yaretzi	Yolanda	Yvonne
Yara	Yasmin	Ysabel	
Yareli	Yasmine	Yvette	

Z NAMES

Zahra	Zara	Zion	Zuri
Zainab	Zaylee	Zoe	
Zaniyah	Zelda	Zoey	

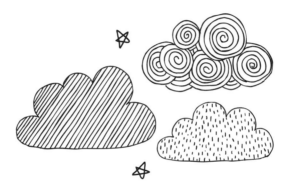

700 GIRLS' NAMES

A

Aaliyah (Arabic) An ascender, one having the highest social standing *Aaleyah, Aaliya, Alea, Aleah, Alee, Aleeya, Aleiya, Alia, Alieya, Aliya, Aliyah, Aliyiah, Alliyia, Alliyah*

Abigail (Hebrew) The source of a father's joy *Abagail, Abbagail, Abbegale, Abbey, Abbi, Abbie, Abbigail, Abby, Abbygail, Abbygayle, Abigael, Abigale, Abigayle, Abygail, Abygayle*

Abra (Hebrew / Arabic) Feminine form of Abraham; mother of a multitude; mother of nations / lesson; example *Abbra, Abbrah, Abrah, Abri, Abria, Abree*

Abril (Spanish / Portuguese) Form of April, meaning "opening buds of spring"

Adah (Hebrew) Ornament; beautiful addition to the family *Ada, Adaya, Adda*

Addison (English) Daughter of Adam *Addeson, Addisyn, Addyson, Adison, Adisson, Adyson*

Adela (German) Of the nobility; serene; of good humor *Adali, Adele, Adelia, Adelie, Adelina, Adella, Adelle*

Adelaide (German) Of the nobility; serene; of good humor *Adelaid*

Adeline (German) Form of Adela, meaning of the nobility *Adalyn, Adalynn, Adelyn, Adelynn*

Adra (Arabic) One who is chaste; a virgin

Adriana (Greek) Feminine form of Adrian; from the Adriatic Sea region; woman with dark features *Adrea, Adreana, Adreanna, Adria, Adriah, Adriane, Adrianna, Adrianne, Adrie, Adriel, Adriene, Adrienna, Adrienne*

Adrina (Italian) Having great happiness *Adreena, Adreenah, Adrinah, Adrinna, Adryna, Adrynah*

Aileen (Irish / Scottish) Light bearer / from the green meadow *Ailean, Ailein, Ailene, Ailin, Aillen, Ailyn, Alean, Aleane*

Ailis (Irish) One who is noble and kind *Ailesh, Ailisa, Ailise, Ailish, Ailyse*

Ailna (German) One who is sweet and pleasant; of the nobility *Ailne*

Ainsley (Scottish) One's own meadow *Ainslee, Ainslei, Ainslie, Ainsly, Ansley, Aynslee, Aynslie*

Aisha (Arabic / African) Lively / womanly *Aiesha, Ayisha, Myisha*

Alaia (Arabic / Basque) One who is majestic, of high worth / joy *Alaiah, Alaya, Alayah*

Alaina (French) Beautiful and fair woman; dear child *Alainah, Alaine, Alana, Alanah, Alanna, Alannah, Alaney, Alani, Alanie, Alanis, Alanney, Alanni, Alayna, Alayne, Alyn*

Alexa (Greek) Form of Alexandra, meaning "a helper and defender of mankind" *Aleka, Alexia*

Alexandra (Greek) Feminine form of Alexander; a helper and defender of mankind *Alejandra, Aleksandra, Alessandra, Alexandrea, Alexandria, Alexis, Alixandra, Alondra, Sandra, Sandrine, Sasha*

Alexis (Greek) Form of Alexandra, meaning "a helper and defender of mankind" *Alexia, Alexus, Alexys*

Ali (English) Form of Allison or Alice, meaning "woman of the nobility" *Alie, Alli, Allie, Ally*

Alice (German) Woman of the nobility; truthful; having high moral character *Aleece, Alesia, Allie, Ally, Alyce*

·········· **Alice** ··········

I knew I wanted a name for my daughter that had some kind of literary tie-in. Classic and elegant, clear but not too obvious... Alice was the perfect choice! —Anna, IL

Alicia (Spanish) Form of Alice, meaning "woman of the nobility" *Alecia, Aleecia, Aleesha, Alesha, Alisa, Alisha, Aliza*

Alina (Arabic / Polish) One who is noble / one who is beautiful and bright *Aleena, Alena, Aline, Alyna*

Allison (English) Form of Alice, meaning "woman of the nobility, truthful; having high moral character" *Alicen, Alisanne, Alisen, Alison, Alisyn, Allisson, Allyson, Alyson*

Alma (Latin / Italian) One who is nurturing and kind / refers to the soul *Almah*

Alpha (Greek) The firstborn child; the first letter of the Greek alphabet

Alyssa (German) Form of Alice, meaning "woman of the nobility, truthful; having high moral character" *Alisa, Alisia, Alishya, Alissa, Alissya, Allisa, Allyssa, Alysa, Alyssaya, Alysse, Alyssia*

Amada (Spanish) One who is loved by all *Amadah, Amadea, Amadia, Amadita*

Amalia (German) One who is industrious and hardworking *Amalea, Amalie, Amalya, Amelia, Amilia, Amyleah, Amylia, Neneca*

Amari (African) Having great strength, a builder *Amaree, Amarie*

Amber (French) Resembling the jewel; a warm honey color *Ambar, Amberlee, Amberli, Amberly, Amberlyn, Ambur, Ambyr, Ambyre*

Amelia (German) Form of Amalia or (Latin) form of Emily, meaning "one who is industrious and hardworking" *Amelie, Amelita, Amely, Amylia*

America (Latin) A powerful ruler *Americus, Amerika, Amerikus*

Amina (Arabic) A princess, one who commands; truthful, trustworthy *Ameera, Ameerah, Ameira, Ameirah, Amiera, Amirah, Amyra, Amyrah*

Amiyah (American) Form of Amy, meaning "dearly loved" *Amiah, Amiya, Amya*

Amy (Latin) Dearly loved *Aimee, Aimey, Aimi, Aimie, Aimy, Aimya, Amice, Amicia*

Anastasia (Greek) One who shall rise again *Anastascia, Anastase, Anastasha, Anastasie, Stacey, Stacia, Stacy, Stasia*

Andrea (Greek / Latin) Courageous and strong / feminine form of Andrew; womanly *Andera, Andreana, Andreia, Andreina, Andreya, Andria, Andriana, Andrianna*

Angel (Greek) A heavenly
messenger

Angela (Greek) A heavenly
messenger; an angel *Angelica,
Angie, Angelina, Angeline,
Angelique, Angelita, Angella,
Angy, Anjela, Anjelika*

Angelina (Greek) Form of
Angela, meaning "a heavenly
messenger; an angel" *Angelene,
Angelin, Angeline, Angelyn*

Anna (Latin) A woman graced
with God's favor *Ana, Ancina,
Ane, Anika, Ann, Annah, Annchen,
Anne, Annie, Annika, Anouche,
Anya*

Annabel (Italian) A graceful
and beautiful woman *Anabel,
Anabell, Anabella, Anabelle,
Annabele, Annabell, Annabella,
Annabelle*

Annalynn (English) From the
graceful lake *Analin, Analine,
Analyn, Analynn, Annalin,
Annaline, Annalinn, Annalyn*

Annmarie (English) Filled
with bitter grace *Anamari,
Anamaria, Anamarie, Annamaria,
Annamarie, Annemaria,
Annemarie, Annmaria*

Antoinette (French)
Praiseworthy *Toinette*

Anya (Russian) Form of Anna,
meaning "a woman graced
with God's favor"

April (English) Opening buds of spring; born in the month of April *Abrielle, Abrienda, Aprel, Aprele, Aprial, Aprila, Aprile, Aprili, Aprielle, Aprilla, Aprille, Apryl, Apryle, Apryll, Aprylle, Averel, Averil, Averill, Averyl, Avrial, Avriel, Avrielle, Avril, Avrill, Avryl*

Arabella (Latin) An answered prayer; beautiful altar *Arabel, Arabela, Arabell*

Arden (Latin / English) One who is passionate and enthusiastic / from the valley of the eagles *Ardan, Ardean, Ardeen, Ardena, Ardene, Ardin, Ardine, Ardun*

Aria (English) A beautiful melody *Ariah*

Ariana (Welsh / Greek) Resembling silver / one who is holy *Aerian, Aerion, Arian, Ariane, Arianie, Arianna, Arianne, Arieon, Aryana, Aryanna*

Ariel (Hebrew) A lionness of God *Airial, Areli, Arely, Ari, Arial, Ariela, Ariele, Arieli, Ariella, Arielle, Ariely, Aryela*

Arin (English) Form of Erin, meaning "woman of Ireland" *Aryn*

Armani (Persian) One who is desired *Armahni, Armanee, Armaney, Armanie*

Arya (Indian) One who is noble and honored *Aryah, Aryana, Aryanna, Aryia*

Ashley (English) From the meadow of ash trees *Ashala, Ashleay, Ashlee, Ashleigh, Ashleye, Ashlie, Ashly, Ashlya*

Ashlyn (American) Combination of Ashley and Lynn *Ashlynn, Ashlynne*

Asia (Greek / English) Resurrection / the rising sun; in the Koran, the woman who raised Moses; a woman from the east

Aspen (English) From the aspen tree *Aspin, Aspina, Aspine, Aspyn, Aspyna, Aspyne*

Astrid (Scandinavian / German) One with divine strength *Astryd, Estrid*

Aubrey (English) One who rules with elf wisdom *Aubree, Aubri, Aubriana, Aubrie, Aubry*

Audrey (English) Woman with noble strength *Adrey, Audra, Audray, Audre, Audrea, Audree, Audrin, Audrina, Audry*

Augusta (Latin) Feminine form of Augustus; venerable, majestic *Agostina, Agostine, Agustina, Agusta, Augusteen, Augustina, Augustine, Augustyna*

Aurora (Latin) Morning's first light; in mythology, the goddess of the dawn *Aurea, Aurore, Aurorette*

Autumn (English) Born in the fall *Autum*

Ava

We had liked Ava for some time, but by the time I was pregnant, the name had skyrocketed in popularity. We searched for other options, thinking that she might want a unique name. But we couldn't find anything we thought was as beautiful and perfect for our baby, and it seemed silly not to choose Ava just because other people loved it too. —Shana, IL

Ava (German / Iranian) A birdlike woman / from the water *Avah, Avalee, Avaleigh, Avaley, Avali, Avalie, Avalynn, Avelaine, Avelina, Ayva*

Avery (English) One who is a wise ruler; of the nobility *Averea, Avereah, Averee, Averey, Averi, Averie, Avrie*

Aviva (Hebrew) One who is innocent and joyful; resembling springtime *Aviv, Avivah, Avivi, Avivice, Avivie, Avni, Avri, Avyva*

Ayanna (Hindi / African) One who is innocent / resembling a beautiful flower *Ahyana, Aiyana, Aiyanna, Anyaniah, Ayana, Ayania, Ayannah, Ayna*

Ayla (Hebrew) From the oak tree *Aileen, Aylah, Aylana, Aylanna, Aylea, Aylee, Ayleen, Ayleena, Aylena, Aylene, Aylin, Ayline*

Aza (Arabic / African) One who provides comfort / powerful *Aiza, Aizha, Aizia, Azia*

B

Bailey (English) From the courtyard within castle walls; a public official *Bailee, Baileigh, Baili, Bailie, Baylee, Bayleigh, Bayley, Baylie*

Barbara (Latin) A traveler from a foreign land; a stranger *Babette, Baibin, Bairbre, Barb, Barbarella, Barbarita, Barbary, Barbra*

Beatrice (Latin) One who blesses others *Bea, Beatricia, Beatrisa, Beatriss, Beatrisse, Beatrix, Beatriz, Beatrize*

Belen (Spanish) Woman from Bethlehem

Belinda (English) A beautiful and tender woman *Balynda, Balyndah, Belienda, Belindah, Belynda, Belyndah, Bleiendah*

Bella (Italian) A woman famed for her beauty *Bela, Belia, Belita, Bell, Bellanca, Bellany, Belle, Bellissa*

Bethany (Hebrew) From the house of figs *Bethan, Bethane, Bethanee, Bethaney, Bethani, Bethanie, Bethann, Bethanne*

Beyonce (American) One who surpasses others *Beyoncay, Beyoncea, Beyoncée, Beyonci, Beyoncie, Beyonsae, Beyonsai, Beyonsay*

Bianca (Italian) A shining, fair-skinned woman *Bianka, Byanca, Byanka*

Billie (English) Feminine form of William; having a desire to protect *Billea, Billeah, Billee, Billeigh, Billey, Billi, Billy*

Blair (Scottish) From the field of battle *Blaer, Blaere, Blaire, Blare, Blayr, Blayre*

Blake (English) A dark beauty *Blaek, Blaeke, Blaik, Blaike, Blayk, Blayke*

Bonnie (English) Pretty face *Bona, Bonea, Boneah, Bonee, Boni*

Braelyn (American) Combination of Braden and Lynn *Braelen, Braelin, Braylen, Braylin, Braylyn*

Brenda (Irish) Feminine form of Brendan; a princess; wielding a sword *Breandan, Brend, Brendalynn, Brendolyn, Brienda, Brinda, Brynda*

Brenna (Irish) A raven-like woman *Bren, Brena, Brenah, Brenn, Brennah, Brina, Brinna*

······· **Brenna** ·······

We chose the name Brenna for my Irish heritage, and also because my husband and I and our two daughters all loved it. We have been surprised at how often she gets called Breanna though. It means "raven," but ironically she has very blond hair! —Nancy, NC

Brianna (Irish) Feminine form of Brian; from the high hill; one who ascends *Breana, Breann, Breanna, Breanne, Breeana, Breeanna, Breona, Breonna, Briana, Bryana, Bryanna*

Brice (Welsh) One who is alert; ambitious *Bryce*

Bridget (Irish) A strong and protective woman; in mythology, goddess of fire, wisdom, and poetry *Birgit, Birgitte, Bridgett, Bridgette, Bridgit, Bridgitte, Briget, Brigette*

Brie (French) Type of cheese *Bree, Breeyah, Bria, Briah, Briya, Briyah, Brya*

Brielle (French) Form of Brie, meaning "type of cheese"

Bristol (English) From the city in England *Bristow, Brystol, Brystow*

Brittany (English) A woman from Great Britain *Britany, Britnee, Britney, Britny, Brittanee, Brittaney, Brittani, Brittanie*

Brook (English) From the running stream *Brooke, Brookie*

Brooklyn (American) Borough of New York City *Brooklin, Brooklynn, Brooklynne*

Brylee (American) Form of Riley, meaning "from the rye clearing; a courageous woman" *Brilee, Briley, Bryli, Brylie*

Brynley (English) From the burnt meadow *Brinley, Brinli, Brynlee, Brynlie, Brynly*

Brynn (Welsh) Hill *Brin, Brinley, Brinli, Brynlie, Brinn, Bryn, Brynlee, Brynly*

C

Cadence (Latin) Rhythmic and melodious; a musical woman *Cadena, Cadencia, Cadenza, Cadian, Cadianne, Cadiene, Cadienne, Caydence, Kadence, Kaydence*

Caia (Latin) One who rejoices *Cai, Cais*

Cailyn (Gaelic) A young woman *Cailin*

Caitlin (English) Form of Catherine, meaning "one who is pure; virginal" *Caitlan, Caitlinn, Caitlyn, Caitlynn, Catlin, Catline, Catlyn*

Calais (French) From the city in France

Calista (Greek) Most beautiful; in mythology, a nymph who changed into a bear and then into the Great Bear constellation *Calissa, Calisto, Calixte, Callista, Calyssa, Calysta, Colista, Collista*

Calla (Greek) Resembling a lily; a beautiful woman *Callah*

Callie (Greek) A beautiful girl *Cali, Callee, Kali, Kallie*

Cameron (Scottish) Having a crooked nose *Camerin, Cameryn, Camren, Camrin, Camron, Camryn*

Camila (Italian) Feminine form of Camillus; a ceremonial attendant; a noble virgin *Caimile, Cam, Camelai, Camile, Camilla, Camille, Camillei, Camillia*

Cara (Italian / Gaelic) One who is dearly loved / a good friend *Carah, Caralee, Caralie, Caralyn, Caralynn, Carra, Carrah, Chara*

Carina (Latin) Little darling *Cariana, Cariena, Carine, Carinna, Caryna, Carinna, Carynna*

Carissa (Greek) A woman of grace *Carisa, Carissima, Carrisa, Carrissa*

Carla (Latin) Feminine form of Carl; a free woman *Carlah, Carlana, Carleen, Carlena, Carlene, Carletta*

Carly (American) Form of Carla, meaning "a free woman" *Carlee, Carleigh, Carley, Carli, Carlie*

Carmel (Hebrew) Of the fruitful orchid *Carmela, Carmella, Karmel*

Carmen (Latin) A beautiful song *Carma, Carmelita, Carmencita, Carmia, Carmie, Carmina, Carmine, Carmita*

Carol (English) Form of Caroline, meaning "joyous song"; feminine form of Charles; a small, strong woman *Carola, Carole, Carolee, Caroli, Carolie, Carolla, Carolle, Caroly*

Caroline (Latin) Joyous song; feminine form of Charles; a small, strong woman *Carol, Carolann, Carolanne, Carolena, Carolene, Caroliana, Carolina, Carolyn*

Carrington (English) A beautiful woman; a woman of Carrington *Carington, Carryngton, Caryngton*

Carys (Welsh) One who loves and is loved *Caris, Cariss, Carisse, Caryss, Carysse, Cerys, Ceryss, Cerysse*

Casey (Greek / Irish) A vigilant woman *Casie, Casy, Caysie, Kasey*

Carson (Scottish) Son of the marshland *Carsan, Carsen, Carsin, Carsyn*

····················· **Carson** ·····················

I liked Carson for a girl and Carter for a boy. My husband loved both names, but vice versa. After a challenging labor in which the epidural refused to commit, a peanut of a girl was born, and out of exasperation I said, "Now can I name this baby?!" My husband couldn't really say no. —Beth, IA

Cassandra (Greek) An unheeded prophetess; in mythology, King Priam's daughter who foretold the fall of Troy *Casandra, Cass, Cassandrea, Cassaundra, Cassey, Cassi, Cassie, Cassondra, Cassy*

Cassidy (Irish) Curly-haired girl *Casidhe, Cassadea, Cassadee, Cassadi, Cassadie, Cassady, Cassidea, Cassidee, Cassidey, Cassidi, Cassidie*

Catherine (English) One who is pure; virginal *Catalina, Catharine, Catherin, Catheryn, Catheryna, Cathi, Cathrine, Cathryn, Cathy, Katherine*

Cecilia (Latin) Feminine form of Cecil; one who is blind; patron saint of music *Cecelia, Cicely, Cecile, Cecilee, Cecily, Cecille, Cecilie, Cicilia, Celia, Sheila, Silka, Sissy*

Celeste (Latin) A heavenly daughter *Celesta, Celestia, Celestina, Celestine, Celestyna, Celisse*

Chana (Hebrew) Form of Hannah, meaning "having favor and grace" *Chaanach, Chaanah, Chanach, Chanah, Channa, Channah*

Chanel (French) From the canal; a channel *Chanell, Chanelle, Channelle, Chenel, Chenell, Chenelle*

Charity (Latin) A woman of generous love *Charitee, Charitey, Chariti, Charitie*

Charlie (English) Form of Charles, meaning "one who is strong" *Charlaine, Charlee, Charlena, Charlene, Charley, Charli, Charlisa, Charlize, Charlyn*

Charlotte (French) Form of Charles, meaning "a small, strong woman" *Charlize, Charlot, Charlotta*

Chelsea (English) From the landing place for chalk *Chelcie, Chelsa, Chelsee, Chelseigh, Chelsey, Chelsi, Chelsie, Chelsy*

Chenille (American) A soft-skinned woman *Chenil, Chenila, Chenile, Chenill, Chenilla*

Cherish (English) To be held dear, valued

Cherry (English) Resembling a fruit-bearing tree *Cherrea, Cherreah, Cherree, Cherrey, Cherri, Cherrie*

Chesney (English) One who promotes peace *Chesnea, Chesneah, Chesnee, Chesni, Chesnie, Chesny*

Cheyenne (Native American) Unintelligible speaker *Chayanne, Cheyane, Cheyene, Shayan, Shyann*

Chiara (Italian) Daughter of the light *Chiarah, Chiarra, Chiarrah*

Chloe (Greek) A flourishing woman; blooming *Chloë, Clo, Cloe, Cloey*

Christina (English) Follower of Christ *Cairistiona, Christal, Christian, Christiana, Christiane, Christianna, Christin, Christinah, Christine, Chrystal, Cristal, Cristine, Crystal, Kristina*

Ciara (Irish) A dark beauty *Ceara, Ciar, Ciaran, Ciarda, Ciarra, Ciera, Ciere, Cierra*

Claire (French) Form of Clara, meaning "one who is famously bright" *Clair, Clare*

Clara (Latin) One who is famously bright *Claire, Clarabelle, Clarice, Clarie, Clarinda, Clarine, Clarrie, Clarry, Clarita, Claritza*

Claudia (Latin / German / Italian) One who is lame *Claudelle, Gladys*

Clementine (French) Feminine form of Clement; one who is merciful *Clem, Clemence, Clemency, Clementia, Clementina, Clementya, Clementyn, Clementyna*

Colette (French) Victory of the people *Collette, Kolette*

Comfort (English) One who strengthens or soothes others *Comforte, Comforteena, Comforteene, Comfortena, Comfortene, Comfortiene, Comfortyna, Comfortyne*

Contessa (Italian) A titled woman; a countess *Contesa, Contesse, Countesa, Countess, Countessa*

Cooper (English) One who makes barrels *Couper*

Cora (English) A young maiden *Corah, Coraline, Corra*

Cordelia (Latin) A good-hearted woman; a woman of honesty *Cordee, Cordelea, Cordella, Cordi, Cordie, Cordilea, Cordilia, Cordy*

Corey (Irish) From the hollow; of the churning waters *Cori, Coriann, Corrianna, Corianne, Corie, Corri, Corrie, Cory*

Corina (Latin) A spear-wielding woman *Corienne, Corine, Corinna, Corinne, Corrinne, Corryn, Coryn, Corynna*

Cornelia (Latin) Feminine form of Cornelius; referring to a horn *Cornalia, Corneelija, Cornela, Cornelija, Cornella, Cornelle, Cornelya, Cornie*

Courtney (English) A courteous woman; courtly *Cordney, Cordni, Cortenay, Corteney, Cortland, Cortnee, Cortneigh, Cortney, Courteney*

Cynthia (Greek) Moon goddess *Cinda, Cindia, Cindy, Cinthea, Cinthia*

D

> ···················· **Dahlia** ····················
>
> We named our daughter Dahlia because it means "small branch" in Hebrew—and she was the first branch for our new family tree. We still love it today, and she gets compliments almost every time someone asks her name. —Ruthie, Montreal

Dahlia (Swedish) From the valley; resembling the flower *Dahiana, Dahl, Dahlea, Daleia, Dalia, Dayha*

Daisy (English) Of the day's eye; resembling a flower *Daisee, Daisey, Daisi, Daisie, Daizy, Dasie, Daysi, Deysi*

Dakota (Native American) A friend to all *Dakoda, Dakodah, Dakotah, Dakotta*

Damani (American) Of a bright tomorrow *Damanea, Damaneah, Damanee, Damaney, Damanie, Damany*

Dana (English) Woman from Denmark *Daena, Daina, Danaca, Danah, Dane, Danet, Daney, Dania, Danna*

Danica (Slavic) Of the morning star *Danika*

Daniela (Spanish) Form of Danielle, meaning "God is my judge" *Daniella*

Danielle (Hebrew) Feminine form of Daniel; God is my judge *Daanelle, Danee, Danele, Danella, Danelle, Danelley, Danette, Daney*

Danna (American) Form of Dana, meaning "woman from Denmark" *Dannah*

Daphne (Greek) Of the laurel tree; in mythology, a virtuous woman transformed into a laurel tree to protect her from Apollo *Daffi, Daffie, Daffy, Dafna, Daphna, Daphney, Daphni, Daphnie*

Darby (English) Of the deer park *Darb, Darbee, Darbey, Darbie, Darrbey, Darrbie, Darrby, Derby, Larby*

Daria (Greek) Feminine form of Darius; possessing good fortune; wealthy *Dari, Darian, Dariane, Darianna, Dariele, Darielle, Darien, Darienne*

Dawn (English) Born at daybreak; of the day's first light *Dawna, Dawne, Dawnelle, Dawnetta, Dawnette, Dawnielle, Dawnika, Dawnita*

Daya (Hebrew) Resembling a bird of prey *Dayah, Dayana, Dayanara, Dayanea, Dayaneah, Dayania, Dayaniah*

Deborah (Hebrew)
Resembling a bee; in the Bible,
a prophetess *Debbera, Debbey,*
Debbi, Debbie, Debbra, Debby

Deidre (Gaelic) A broken-
hearted or raging woman
Deadra, Dede, Dedra, Deedra,
Deedre, Deidra, Deirdre, Deidrie

Delaney (Irish / French)
The dark challenger / from
the elder-tree grove *Delaina,*
Delaine, Delainey, Delainy,
Delane, Delanie, Delany, Delayna

Delilah (Hebrew) A seductive
woman *Delila, Delyla, Delylah*

Demi (Greek) A petite woman
Demea, Demee, Demiana,
Demianna, Demianne, Demie,
Demy

Denise (French) Feminine
form of Dennis; a follower
of Dionysus *Denese, Denice,*
Deniece, Denisa, Denissa, Denize,
Denyce, Denys, Denyse

Desiree (French) One who
is desired *Desarae, Desaree,*
Desirae, Desirat, Desire, Desyre,
Dezirae, Deziree

Destiny (English)
Recognizing one's certain
fortune; fate *Destanee, Destina,*
Destine, Destinee, Destiney,
Destini, Destinie, Destyni

Diana (Latin) Of the divine;
in mythology, goddess of the
moon and the hunt *Dayana,*
Dayanna, Deanna, Dianna

Diane (Latin) Form of Diana, meaning "of the divine" *Dayann, Dayanne, Deana, Deandra, Deane, Deann*

Dixie (English) Woman from the South *Dixee, Dixey, Dixi, Dixy*

Dolores (Spanish) Woman of sorrow; refers to the Virgin Mary *Dalores, Delora, Delores, Deloria, Deloris, Dolorcita, Dolorcitas, Dolorita*

Dominique (French) Feminine form of Dominic; born on the Lord's day *Domaneke, Domanique, Domenica, Domeniga, Domenique, Dominee, Domineek, Domineke*

Dorothy (Greek) A gift of God *Dasha, Dasya, Dodie, Dody, Doe, Doll, Dolley, Dolli*

Dulce (Latin) A very sweet woman *Dulcee, Dulcie, Dulcina*

Dylan (Welsh) Daughter of the waves *Dillan, Dillen, Dillian, Dillon, Dylana, Dylane, Dyllan, Dyllana*

E

Ebony (Egyptian) A dark beauty *Ebonea, Eboneah, Ebonee, Eboney, Eboni, Ebonie, Ebonique*

Eden (Hebrew) Place of pleasure *Edan, Edin, Edon*

Edith (English) The spoils of war; one who is joyous; a treasure *Eda, Edalyn, Edalynn, Edee, Edelina, Edeline, Edelyne, Edelynn, Edie, Edita, Edyta, Edyth, Eydie*

Edna (Hebrew) One who brings pleasure; a delight *Ednah, Edena, Edenah*

Eileen (Gaelic) Form of Evelyn, meaning "a birdlike woman" *Eila, Eilean, Eileene, Eilena, Eilene, Eilin, Eilleen, Eily*

Elaine (French) Form of Helen, meaning "the shining light" *Elaena, Elaene, Elaina, Elayna, Elayne, Ellaina, Ellaine, Ellayne*

Elana (Hebrew) From the oak tree *Elan, Elanah, Elanee, Elaney, Elani, Elanie, Elanna, Elany*

Eleanor (Greek) Form of Helen, meaning "the shining light" *Eleanora, Eleanore, Eleni, Eleonora, Eleonore, Elinor, Elinora, Elnora, Nora*

Elena (Spanish) Form of Helen, meaning "the shining light" *Eleena, Eleenah, Elenah, Eleni, Eliana, Elina, Elinah, Elyna, Elynah*

Eliana (Hebrew) The Lord answers our prayers *Eleana, Elia, Eliane, Eliann, Elianna, Elianne, Elyan, Elyana, Elyann, Elyanna, Elyanne*

Elisa (English) Form of Elizabeth, meaning "my God is bountiful" *Elisha, Elishia, Elisia, Elissa, Elysa, Elysha, Elysia, Elyssa*

Elise (English) Form of Elizabeth, meaning "my God is bountiful" *Elice, Elisse, Elle, Elyse, Elysse, Ilyse*

Elizabeth (Hebrew) My God is bountiful; God's promise *Babette, Beth, Elisabet, Elisabeth, Elisabetta, Elissa, Eliza, Elizabel, Elizabet, Elsa, Ilsabet, Ilsabeth, Itzel, Libby, Lisa, Liz*

Ella (German) From a foreign land *Ela, Elle, Ellee, Ellesse, Elli, Ellia, Ellie, Elly*

Ellen (English) Form of Helen, meaning "the shining light" *Elen, Elynn, Elin, Elleen, Ellena, Ellene, Ellin, Ellyn*

Elliana (Hebrew) Form of Eliana, meaning "the Lord answers our prayers"

Ellie (English) Form of Eleanor, meaning "the shining light" *Elleigh, Elley, Elli, Elly*

Eloisa (Latin) Form of Louise, meaning "a famous warrior" *Aloisa, Aloise, Eloise, Eloisee, Eloiza, Eloize, Eloizee*

Elsie (English) Form of Elizabeth, meaning "my God is bountiful"

Emelia

We named our daughter Emelia Margaret after a great-aunt and her grandmother (and we found out later that her paternal great-great grandmothers were named Emelia and Margaret). We wanted a traditional name yet something not found on any top 100 list so there wouldn't be ten other girls with the same name in her class. —Meghan, WA

Ember (English) A low-burning fire *Embar, Embir, Embyr*

Emerson (German) Offspring of Emery *Emmerson, Emyrson*

Emery (German) Industrious *Emeri, Emerie, Emori, Emorie, Emory*

Emily (Latin) An industrious and hardworking woman *Emeleigh, Emeli, Emelia, Emelie, Emely, Emilee, Emileigh, Emilia, Emilie, Emmalee*

Emma (German) One who is complete; a universal woman *Emelina, Emeline, Emmajean, Emmalee, Emmaline, Emmi, Emmie, Emmy*

Emmylou (American) A universal ruler *Emilou, Emielou, Emmielou, Emmilou, Emylou*

Enslie (American) An emotional woman *Ensli, Ensley, Ensly, Enslee, Enslea, Ensleigh*

Erica (Scandinavian / Latin) Feminine form of Eric; ever the ruler / resembling heather *Eiric, Ericca, Ericka, Erics, Erika, Erike, Erikka, Eryka, Rica*

Erin (Gaelic) Woman from Ireland *Arin, Erienne, Erina, Erinn, Erinna, Erinne, Eryn, Eryna, Erynn*

Esme (French) An esteemed woman *Esmai, Esmae, Esmay, Esmaye, Esmee*

Esther (Persian) Resembling the myrtle leaf *Eistir, Ester, Eszter, Eszti*

Estrella (Spanish) Star *Estrela*

Eugenia (Greek) A well-born woman *Eugenie, Gina, Zenechka*

Eva (Hebrew) Giver of life; a lively woman *Eeva, Eve, Evetta, Evette, Evia, Eviana, Evie, Evita*

Evangeline (Greek) A bringer of good news *Evangelina, Evangelyn*

Evelyn (German) A birdlike woman *Eileen, Evaleen, Evalina, Evaline, Evalyn, Evelin, Evelina, Eveline, Evelyne, Evelynn*

Everly (English) Boar in a wild field *Everlee, Everleigh, Everley, Everlie*

Evline (French) One who loves nature *Evlean, Evleane, Evleen, Evleene, Evlene, Evlyn, Evlyne*

F

Faith (English) Having a belief and trust in God *Faithe, Faithful, Fayana, Fayane, Fayanna, Fayanne, Fayth, Faythe*

Fallon (Irish) A commanding woman *Faleen, Faleene, Falina, Faline, Falinne, Fallyn, Falyn, Falynne*

Fatima (Arabic) The perfect woman *Fahima, Fahimah, Fatimah*

Fay (English) From the fairy kingdom; a fairy or an elf *Fae, Fai, Faie, Faye, Fayette, Faylinn, Faylyn, Faylynn*

Felicity (Latin) Form of Felicia, meaning "happy" *Felicie, Felicy, Felisa*

Fernanda (Spanish) Feminine form of Fernando; an adventurous woman

Filipa (Spanish) Feminine form of Phillip; a friend of horses *Filipah, Filipeena, Filipina, Filippa, Filipyna, Fillipa, Fillippa*

Fina (English) Feminine form of Joseph; God will add *Feana, Feena, Fifine, Fifna, Fifne, Finah, Fini, Fyna*

Finley (Gaelic) A fair-haired hero *Fin, Finlay, Finlee, Finli, Finlie, Finly, Finn, Finnlee, Finnley, Finnli*

Fiona (Gaelic) One who is fair; a white-shouldered woman *Finna, Fionavar, Fione, Fionn, Fionna, Fionnghuala, Fionnuala, Fynballa*

Florence (Latin) A flourishing woman; a blooming flower *Florencia, Florenteena, Florenteene, Florentina, Florentine, Florentyna, Florentyne, Florenza*

Forest (English) A woodland dweller *Forrest*

Forever (American) Everlasting

Francesca (Italian) Form of Frances, meaning "one who is free" *Fran, Frances, Franchesca, Francia, Francie, Francina, Francisca*

Frederica (German) Peaceful ruler *Freda, Freddie, Freida, Rica*

Freira (Spanish) A sister *Freirah, Freyira, Freyirah*

Fran

We named our girl Fran Dandelion. We liked the old-world simplicity of Fran, plus it makes me think of a rolling meadow. The Dandelion just belongs in that meadow, plus it touches a cute/hippie nerve in us. We now think all our kids' names will have some kind of plant or grain in them (Thistle, Rye...).
—Ilana, TX

Freya (Norse) A lady *Freja, Freyah, Freyja*

Frida (German) Peaceful *Frieda, Fryda*

Fuchsia (Latin) Resembling the flower *Fewshea, Fewshia, Fewsha, Fusha, Fushea, Fushia*

G

Gabriella (Italian / Spanish) Feminine form of Gabriel; heroine of God *Gabriela, Gabriellia, Gabrila, Gabryela, Gabryella*

Gabrielle (Hebrew) Feminine form of Gabriel; heroine of God *Gabriel, Gabriela, Gabriele, Gabriell, Gabriellen, Gabriellia, Gabrila*

Gemma (Latin) As precious as a jewel *Gem, Gema, Gemmaline, Gemmalyn, Gemmalynn, Jemma*

Genesis (Hebrew) Of the beginning; the first book of the Bible *Genesies, Genesiss, Genessa, Genisis*

Genevieve (French) White wave; fair-skinned *Genavieve, Geneve, Genevie, Genivee, Genivieve, Gennie, Genny, Genoveva*

Georgia (Greek) Feminine form of George; one who works the earth; a farmer; from the state of Georgia *Georgeann, Georgeanne, Georgena, Georgene, Georgetta, Georgette, Georgiana, Georgina, Jeorjia*

Gertrude (German) Adored warrior *Geertruide, Geltruda, Geltrudis, Gert, Gerta, Gerte, Gertie, Gertina, Trudy*

Gia (Italian) Form of Gianna, meaning "God is gracious" *Giah*

Gianna (Italian) Feminine form of John, meaning "God is gracious" *Gia, Giana, Giovana*

Gillian (Latin) One who is youthful *Ghilian, Gilian, Giliana, Gillianne*

Gina (Japanese / English) A silvery woman / form of Eugenia, meaning "a well-born woman"; form of Jean, meaning "God is gracious" *Geana, Geanndra, Geena, Geina, Gena, Genalyn, Geneene, Genelle*

Ginger (English) A lively woman; resembling the spice *Gingea, Gingee, Gingey, Gingi, Gingie, Gingy, Ginjer*

Ginny (English) Form of Virginia, meaning "one who is chaste; virginal" *Ginna, Ginnee, Ginnelle, Ginnette, Ginney, Ginni, Ginnie, Ginnilee*

Giselle (French) One who offers her pledge *Gisel, Gisela, Gisella, Jiselle*

Gita (Hindi / Hebrew) A beautiful song / a good woman *Gatha, Gayatri, Geeta, Geetah, Gitah, Gitel, Gitika, Gittell*

Giulia (Italian) Form of Julia, meaning "one who is youthful; daughter of the sky" *Giuliana, Giulie, Giulietta, Giuliette*

Gloria (Latin) A renowned and highly praised woman *Gloree, Gloriana, Gloriane, Glorianna, Glorie, Glorya*

Grace (Latin) Having God's favor; in mythology, the Graces were the personification of beauty, charm, and grace *Gracee, Gracella, Gracelyn, Gracelynn, Gracelynne, Gracey, Gracia, Graciana, Gracie*

Gracie (Latin) Form of Grace, meaning "having God's favor" *Gracee, Gracey, Graci*

Greer (Scottish) Feminine form of Gregory; one who is alert and watchful *Grear, Grier, Gryer*

Greta (German) Resembling a pearl *Greeta, Gretal, Gretchen, Grete, Gretel, Gretha, Grethe, Grethel, Gretna*

Guadalupe (Spanish) From the valley of wolves *Guadelupe, Lupe, Lupita*

Guinevere (Welsh) One who is fair; of the white wave; in mythology, King Arthur's queen *Guenever, Guenevere, Gueniver, Guenna, Guennola, Guinever, Guinna, Gwen*

Gwendolyn (Welsh) One who is fair; of the white ring *Guendolen, Guendolin, Guendolinn, Guendolynn, Guenna, Gwen, Gwenda, Gwendaline, Wendy*

Gwyneth (Welsh) One who is blessed with happiness *Gweneth, Gwenith, Gwenyth, Gwineth, Gwinneth, Gwinyth, Gwynith, Gwynna*

H

Hadassah (Hebrew) From the myrtle tree *Hadasa, Hadasah, Hadassa*

Hadley (English) From the field of heather *Hadlea, Hadlee, Hadleigh, Hadly, Hedlea, Hedleigh, Hedley, Hedlie*

Hailey (English) From the field of hay *Haeleigh, Hailee, Haleigh, Haley, Hayle, Haylee, Hayley, Haylie*

Hallie (Scandinavian / Greek / English) From the hall / woman of the sea / from the field of hay *Halle, Hallea, Halleah, Hallee, Halleigh, Halley, Hallie, Hally*

Halo (Latin) Having a blessed aura *Haelo, Hailo, Haylo*

Halsey (American) A playful woman *Halcey, Halcie, Halcy, Halsea, Halsee, Halsi, Halsie, Halsy*

Hana (Japanese / Arabic) Resembling a flower blossom / a blissful woman *Hanah, Hanako*

Hannah (Hebrew) Having favor and grace; in the Bible, mother of Samuel *Chana, Hanalee, Hanalise, Hanna, Hanne, Hannele, Hannelore, Hannie, Hanny*

········· **Hannah** ·········

From the moment of conception I imagined having a daughter named Hannah. When I discussed it with my husband, he responded, "Like Hanna-Barbera, the cartoon people?" Four hours after her birth, Hannah Elizabeth received her name. When we announced it to the family, my father-in-law's response was: "Like Hanna-Barbera..." I responded, "Different spelling." —Maureen, FL

Harley (English) From the meadow of the hares *Harlea, Harlee, Harleen, Harleigh, Harlene, Harli, Harlie, Harly*

Harlow (American) An impetuous woman

Harmony (English / Latin) Unity / musically in tune *Harmonee, Harmoni, Harmonie*

Harper (English) One who plays or makes harps

Harriet (German) Feminine form of Henry; ruler of the house *Hanrietta, Hanriette, Harrette, Harriett, Harrietta, Harriette*

Haven (English) One who provides a safe haven *Haevan, Haeven, Haevin, Havan, Havin, Havon, Havyn, Hayvan, Hayven, Hayvin, Hayvon, Hayvyn*

Hayden (English) From the hedged valley *Haden, Hadyn, Haeden, Haedyn, Haydan, Haydn, Haydon*

Hazel (English) From the hazel tree *Haesel, Haezel, Haizel, Hayzel, Hazal, Hazell, Hazelle, Hazle*

Heather (English) Resembling the evergreen flowering plant *Heath, Heatha, Heathe, Hether*

Heaven (American) From paradise; from the sky *Heavely, Heavenlea, Heavenlee, Heavenleigh, Heavenley, Heavenli, Heavenlie, Heavenly, Heavyn, Heavynne, Hevan, Hevean*

Heidi (German) Of the nobility, serene *Heide, Heidy, Hydie*

Helen (Greek) The shining light; in mythology, Helen was the most beautiful woman in the world *Aleen, Elaine, Eleanor, Elena, Ellen, Galina, Halina, Heirnine, Helaine, Helana, Heleena, Helena, Helene, Helenna, Helice, Hellen, Leanna, Yalena*

Helia (Greek) Daughter of the sun *Helea, Heleah, Heliah, Heliya, Heliyah, Hellar, Heller*

Helma (German) Form of Wilhelmina, meaning "determined protector" *Helmah, Helmea, Helmeena, Helmia, Helmina, Helmine, Helmyna, Helmyne*

Heloise (French) One who is famous in battle *Helois, Heloisa, Helewidis*

Henrietta (German) Feminine form of Henry; ruler of the house *Henretta, Henrieta, Henriette, Henrika, Henryetta, Hetta, Hette, Hettie*

Hilary (Latin) A cheerful woman *Ellery, Hillary, Hillery*

Holly (English) Of the holly tree *Holle, Hollea, Hollee, Holley, Holli, Hollie, Hollyanne, Hollye*

Hope (English) One who has high expectations through faith

I

Ianthe (Greek) Resembling the violet flower; in mythology, a sea nymph, a daughter of Oceanus *Iantha, Ianthia, Ianthina*

Ida (Greek) One who is diligent; hardworking; in mythology, the nymph who cared for Zeus on Mount Ida *Idaea, Idaia, Idalee, Idalia, Idalie, Idana, Idania*

Iliana (English) Form of Aileen, meaning "light bearer" *Ilene, Ilianna, Iline, Ilyana, Ilyanna, Ilyne*

Iman (Arabic) Having great faith *Imaan, Imain, Imaine, Imanea, Imanee, Imaney, Imani, Imania, Imanie, Imany, Imayn*

Imari (Japanese) Daughter of today *Imarea, Imaree, Imarey, Imarie, Imary*

Ingrid (Scandinavian) Having the beauty of the god Ing *Inga, Inge, Inger, Ingmar, Ingrad, Ingred, Ingria, Ingrida, Ingrit, Inkeri*

Inis (Irish) Woman from Ennis *Iniss, Inisse, Innis, Innys, Inys, Inyss, Inysse*

Irene (Greek) A peaceful woman; in mythology, the goddess of peace *Eirene, Ira, Irayna, Ireen, Iren, Irena, Irenea, Irenee, Irenka*

Iris (Greek) Of the rainbow; a flower; a messenger goddess *Irea, Iria, Irida, Iridian, Iridiana, Iridianny, Irisa, Irisha, Iriss, Irita, Irys, Iryss*

Irma (German) A universal woman

Isabel (Spanish) Form of Elizabeth, meaning "my God is bountiful; God's promise" *Isabeau, Isabela, Isabele, Isabelita, Isabell, Isabelle, Ishbel, Ysabel*

Isabella (Italian / Spanish) Form of Isabel, meaning "consecrated to God" *Isabela, Isabelita, Isibela, Isibella, Isobella, Izabella*

Isadore (Greek) A gift from the goddess Isis *Isador, Isadora, Isadoria, Isidor, Isidora, Isidoro, Isidorus, Isidro*

Isla (Gaelic) From the island *Islae, Islai, Isleta*

Isabella

We decided to name our daughter Isabella because her name wasn't on any baby list at the time. Ironically, others must have had the same thought because it's one of the more popular names of that year! We also thought it would be difficult to abbreviate to anything but Bella. Instead, everyone calls her Izzy (which makes us cringe). —Stephanie, IL

Isleen (Gaelic) Form of Aisling, meaning "a dream or vision; an inspiration" *Isleene, Isleine, Islene, Isleyne, Isliene, Isline, Islyn, Islyne*

Ivory (English) Having a creamy-white complexion; as precious as elephant tusks *Ivorea, Ivoree, Ivoreen, Ivorey, Ivori, Ivorie, Ivorine, Ivoryne*

Isolde (Celtic) A woman known for her beauty; in mythology, the lover of Tristan *Iseult, Iseut, Isold, Isolda, Isolt, Isolte, Isota, Isotta*

Ivy (English) Resembling the evergreen vining plant *Ivea, Ivi, Ivie*

Ivana (Slavic) Feminine form of Ivan; God is gracious *Iva, Ivah, Ivane, Ivanea, Ivania, Ivanka, Ivanna, Ivanne, Ivanya*

J

> ·················· **Jacqueline** ··················
>
> We suspected we were having a boy, so we had settled on a
> boy's name but not a girl's. Of course, we wound up having a
> girl. We stared at her for a while trying to determine who she
> was. We decided she looked like a Jackie. Now she fits her
> name perfectly, although I don't know if she'll ever grow into
> a Jacqueline. —Irene, CA

Jacey (American) Form of Jacinda, meaning "resembling the hyacinth" *Jacee, Jacelyn, Jaci, Jacie, Jacine, Jacy, Jaicee, Jaycee*

Jacqueline (French) Feminine form of Jacques, meaning "the supplanter" *Jacalin, Jacalyn, Jacalynn, Jackalin, Jackalinne, Jackelyn, Jackie, Jacquelyn, Xaquelina*

Jade (Spanish) Resembling the green gemstone *Jadeana, Jadee, Jadine, Jadira, Jadrian, Jadrienne, Jady*

Jamie (Hebrew) Feminine form of James, meaning "she who supplants" *Jaima, Jaime, Jaimee, Jaimelynn, Jaimey, Jaimi, Jaimie, Jaimy*

Jane (Hebrew) Feminine form of John; God is gracious *Jaina, Jaine, Jainee, Jana, Janae, Janaye, Jandy, Janel, Janelle, Janey, Sine*

Janet (Scottish) Feminine form of John, meaning "God is gracious" *Janeta, Janetta, Janette, Janit, Jenetta*

Janis (English) Feminine form of John; God is gracious *Janeece, Janess, Janessa, Janesse, Janessia, Janice, Janicia, Janiece*

Jaslene (American) Form of Jocelyn, meaning "one who is cheerful, happy" *Jaslin, Jaslyn, Jazlyn, Jazlynn*

Jasmine (Persian) Resembling the climbing plant with fragrant flowers *Jaslyn, Jaslynn, Jasmin, Jasmyn, Jazmin, Jazmine, Jazmyn*

Jayda (English) Resembling the green gemstone *Jada, Jaida, Jaidah, Jaydah*

Jayla (Arabic) One who is charitable *Jaela, Jaila, Jaylah, Jaylee, Jayleen, Jaylen, Jaylene, Jaylin, Jaylyn, Jaylynn*

Jean (Hebrew) Feminine form of John; God is gracious *Jeanae, Jeanay, Jeane, Jeanee, Jeanelle, Jeanetta, Jeanette, Jeanice, Gina*

Jemma (English) Form of Gemma, meaning "as precious as a jewel" *Jema, Jemah, Jemalyn, Jemmah, Jemmalyn*

Jennifer

My oldest daughter was three when I was expecting our second child, and when we asked her if it was going to be a boy or a girl, she always said, "It's going to be a girl and we are going to name her Jennifer." After hearing that so often, we got worn down—Jennifer she is. —Diane, IA

Jena (Arabic) Our little bird
Jenah, Jenna

Jennifer (Welsh) One who is fair; a beautiful girl *Jen, Jenefer, Jeni, Jenifer, Jeniffer, Jenn, Jenna, Jennee, Jenni, Jenny*

Jessica (Hebrew) The Lord sees all *Jess, Jessa, Jessaca, Jessaka, Jessalin, Jessalyn, Jesse, Jesseca, Jessie, Yessica*

Jillian (English) Form of Gillian, meaning "one who is youthful" *Jilian, Jiliana, Jill, Jillaine, Jillan, Jillana, Jillane, Jillanne, Jillayne, Jillene, Jillesa, Jilliana, Jilliane, Jilliann, Jillianna*

Jo (English) Feminine form of Joseph, meaning "God will add" *Jobelle, Jobeth, Jodean, Jodelle, Joetta, Joette, Jolinda, Jolisa*

Joanna (French) Feminine form of John, meaning "God is gracious" *Joana*

Jocelyn (German / Latin) From the tribe of Gauts / one who is cheerful, happy *Jocelin, Jocelina, Jocelinda, Joceline, Jocelyne, Jocelynn, Jocelynne, Josalind, Joslyn, Joslynn, Joselyn*

Jolene (English) Feminine form of Joseph, meaning "God will add" *Joeleen, Joeline, Jolaine, Jolean, Joleen, Jolena, Jolina*

Jolie (French) A pretty young woman *Joely, Jolee, Joleigh, Joley, Joli, Joly*

Jordan (Hebrew) Of the downflowing river; in the Bible, the river where Jesus was baptized *Jardena, Johrdan, Jordain, Jordaine, Jordana, Jordane, Jordanka, Jordyn, Jordin*

Josephine (French) Feminine form of Joseph; God will add *Iosepine, Jo, Josefina, Josephene, Josie*

Joy (Latin) A delight; one who brings pleasure to others *Jioia, Jioya, Joi, Joia, Joie, Joya, Joyann, Joyanna*

Joyce (English) One who brings joy to others *Joice, Joyceanne, Joycelyn, Joycelynn, Joyceta, Joyse*

Judith (Hebrew) Woman from Judea *Hudes, Judeana, Judeena, Judit, Judita, Juditha, Judithe, Judyth, Judytha*

Julia (Latin) One who is youthful; daughter of the sky *Jiulia, Joleta, Joletta, Jolette, Julaine, Julayna, Julee, Juleen, Julianne, Julie, Julieta*

Juliana (Spanish) Form of Julia, meaning "one who is youthful" *Julianna*

Juliet (French) Form of Julia, meaning "one who is youthful" *Juliette, Julissa, Julitta*

June (Latin) One who is youthful; born during the month of June *Junae, Junel, Junelle, Junette, Junia, Junita*

Justice (English) One who upholds moral rightness and fairness *Justis, Justise, Justiss, Justus, Justyce, Justyss*

K

Kaelyn (English) A beautiful girl from the meadow *Kaelynn, Kaelynne, Kaelin, Kailyn, Kaylyn, Kaelinn, Kaelinne*

Kaitlyn (Greek) Form of Katherine, meaning "one who is pure; virginal" *Kaitlin, Kaitlan, Kaitleen, Kaitlynn, Katalin, Katalina, Katalyn, Katelin, Kateline, Katelinn, Katelyn, Katelynn, Katilyn, Katlin*

Kala (Arabic / Hawaiian) A moment in time / form of Sarah, meaning "a princess; lady" *Kalah, Kalla, Kallah*

Kallie (English) Form of Callie, meaning "a beautiful girl" *Kalli, Kallita, Kally, Kalley, Kallee, Kalleigh, Kallea, Kalleah*

Kamala (Arabic) A woman of perfection *Kamalah, Kammala, Kamalla*

Kamila (Spanish) Form of Camilla, meaning "a ceremonial attendant" *Kamilah*

Kara (Greek / Italian / Gaelic) One who is pure / dearly loved / a good friend *Karah, Karalee, Karalie, Karalyn, Karalynn, Karrah, Karra, Khara*

Karen (Greek) Form of Katherine, meaning "one who is pure; virginal" *Karan, Karena, Kariana, Kariann, Karianna, Karianne, Karin, Karina*

Karina (Scandinavian / Russian) One who is dear and pure *Karinah, Kareena, Karyna*

Karla (German) Feminine form of Karl; a small, strong woman *Karly, Karli, Karlie, Karleigh, Karlee, Karley, Karlin, Karlyn, Karlina, Karleen*

Kasey (Irish) Form of Casey, meaning "a vigilant woman" *Kacie, Kaci, Kacy, KC, Kacee, Kacey, Kasie, Kasi*

Kate (English) Form of Katherine, meaning "one who is pure; virginal" *Katie, Katey, Kati*

Katherine (Greek) Form of Catherine, meaning "one who is pure; virginal" *Katharine, Katharyn, Kathy, Kathleen, Katheryn, Kathie, Kathrine, Kathryn, Karen, Kay*

Katriel (Hebrew) Crowned by God *Katriele, Katrielle, Katriell*

·········· **Katie** ··········

Our first daughter is Katie Jane. She is not Katherine or Kathleen, because I wanted her "official" first name to be what she was called on a regular basis. But I do end up explaining that it is not a nickname, which kind of defeats the purpose. She also gets called Kate quite often, which frustrates her and me. —Jane, IL

Kay (English / Greek) The keeper of the keys / form of Katherine, meaning "one who is pure; virginal" *Kaye, Kae, Kai, Kaie, Kaya, Kayana, Kayane, Kayanna*

Kayla (Arabic / Hebrew) Crowned with laurel *Kaylah, Kalan, Kalen, Kalin, Kalyn, Kalynn, Kaylan, Kaylana, Kaylin, Kaylen, Kaylynn, Kaylyn, Kayle*

Kaylee (American) Form of Kayla, meaning "crowned with laurel" *Kaleigh, Kaley, Kaelee, Kaeley, Kaeli, Kailee, Kailey, Kalee, Kayleigh, Kayley, Kayli, Kaylie*

Keaton (English) From a shed town *Keatan, Keatyn, Keatin, Keatun*

Keeya (African) Resembling a flower *Keeyah, Kieya, Keiya, Keyya*

Keira (Irish) Form of Kiera, meaning "little dark-haired one" *Kierra, Kyera, Kyerra, Keiranne, Kyra, Kyrie, Kira, Kiran*

Keisha (American) The favorite child; form of Kezia, meaning "of the spice tree" *Keishla, Keishah, Kecia, Kesha, Keysha, Keesha, Kiesha, Keshia*

······································· **Kayla** ·······································

We named our daughter Kayla because the name Kay is so prominent in our family. Her paternal grandmother, maternal grandmother, and myself, her mother, all have the middle name of Kay. —Melissa, IA

Kelly (Irish) A lively and bright-headed woman *Kelley, Kelli, Kellie, Kellee, Kelliegh, Kellye, Keely, Keelie, Keeley, Keelyn*

Kelsey (English) From the island of ships *Kelsie, Kelcey, Kelcie, Kelcy, Kellsie, Kelsa, Kelsea, Kelsee, Kelsi, Kelsy, Kellsey*

Kendall (Welsh) From the royal valley *Kendal, Kendyl, Kendahl, Kindall, Kyndal, Kenley*

Kendra (English) Feminine form of Kendrick; having royal power; from the high hill *Kendrah, Kendria, Kendrea, Kindra, Kindria*

Kenley (American) Form of Kinley and McKinley, meaning "offspring of the fair hero"

Kennedy (Gaelic) A helmeted chief *Kennedi, Kennedie, Kennedey, Kennedee, Kenadia, Kenadie, Kenadi, Kenady, Kenadey*

Kensington (English) A brash lady *Kensyngton, Kensingtyn, Kinsington, Kinsyngton, Kinsingtyn*

Kenzie (American) Diminutive of McKenzie, meaning "daughter of a wise leader; a fiery woman; one who is fair"

Keyla (English) A wise daughter

Khloe (Greek) Form of Chloe, meaning "a flourishing woman; blooming"

Kiara (American) Form of Chiara, meaning "daughter of the light"

Kiley (American) Form of Kylie, meaning "a boomerang"

Kimball (English) Chief of the warriors; possessing royal boldness *Kimbal, Kimbell, Kimbel, Kymball, Kymbal*

Kimberly (English) Of the royal fortress *Kimberley, Kimberli, Kimberlee, Kimberleigh, Kimberlin, Kimberlyn, Kymberlie, Kymberly*

Kimora (American) Form of Kimberly, meaning "of the royal fortress"

Kinley (American) Form of McKinley, meaning "offspring of the fair hero"

Kinsey (English) The king's victory *Kinnsee, Kinnsey, Kinnsie, Kinsee, Kinsie, Kinzee, Kinzie, Kinzey*

Kinsley (English) From the king's meadow *Kinsly, Kinslee, Kinsleigh, Kinsli, Kinslie, Kingsley, Kingslee, Kingslie*

Kristina (English) Form of Christina, meaning "follower of Christ" *Kristena, Kristine, Kristyne, Kristyna, Krystina, Krystine*

Kyla (English) Feminine form of Kyle; from the narrow channel *Kylah, Kylar, Kyle*

Kylie (Australian) A boomerang *Kylee, Kyleigh, Kyley, Kyli, Kyleen, Kyleen, Kyler, Kily, Kileigh, Kilee, Kilie, Kili, Kilea, Kylea*

Kyra (Greek) Form of Cyrus, meaning "noble" *Kyrah, Kyria, Kyriah, Kyrra, Kyrrah*

L

Lacey (French) Woman from Normandy; as delicate as lace *Lace, Lacee, Lacene, Laci, Laciann, Lacie, Lacina, Lacy*

Laila (Arabic) A beauty of the night; born at nightfall *Layla, Laylah*

Laura (Latin) Crowned with laurel; from the laurel tree *Lauraine, Lauralee, Laralyn, Laranca, Larea, Lari, Lauralee, Lauren, Loretta*

Lauren (French) Form of Laura, meaning "crowned with laurel; from the laurel tree" *Laren, Larentia, Larentina, Larenzina, Larren, Laryn, Larryn, Larrynn*

Lauren

Lauren was named in the hospital room after her delivery. I had picked out a boy's name, expecting a boy. On my side table in the hospital was a bottle of Lauren perfume, and that was the name that was chosen. —Lisa, VA

Leah (Hebrew) One who is weary; in the Bible, Jacob's first wife *Leia, Leigha, Lia, Liah, Leeya*

Leanna (Gaelic) Form of Helen, meaning "the shining light" *Leana, Leann, Leanne, Lee-Ann, Leeann, Leeanne, Leianne, Leyanne*

Leila (Persian) Night; dark beauty *Leela, Lela*

Leslie (Gaelic) From the holly garden; of the gray fortress *Leslea, Leslee, Lesleigh, Lesley, Lesli, Lesly, Lezlee, Lezley*

Lia (Italian) Form of Leah, meaning "one who is weary"

Libby (English) Form of Elizabeth, meaning "my God is bountiful; God's promise" *Libba, Libbee, Libbey, Libbie, Libet, Liby, Lilibet, Lilibeth*

Liberty (English) An independent woman; having freedom *Libertey, Libertee, Libertea, Liberti, Libertie, Libertas, Libera, Liber*

Lila (Arabic / Greek) Born at night / resembling a lily *Lilah, Lyla, Lylah*

Lilac (Latin) Resembling the bluish-purple flower *Lilack, Lilak, Lylac, Lylack, Lylak, Lilach*

Lilette (Latin) Resembling a budding lily *Lilett, Lilete, Lilet, Lileta, Liletta, Lylette, Lylett, Lylete*

Liliana (Italian, Spanish) Form of Lillian, meaning "resembling the lily" *Lilliana, Lillianna, Liliannia, Lilyana, Lilia*

Lilith (Babylonian) Woman of the night *Lilyth, Lillith, Lillyth, Lylith, Lyllith, Lylyth, Lyllyth, Lilithe*

Lillian (Latin) Resembling the lily *Lilian, Liliane, Lilianne, Lilias, Lilas, Lillas, Lillias*

Lily (English) Resembling the flower; one who is innocent and beautiful *Leelee, Lil, Lili, Lilie, Lilla, Lilley, Lilli, Lillie, Lilly*

Linda (Spanish) One who is soft and beautiful *Lindalee, Lindee, Lindey, Lindi, Lindie, Lindira, Lindka, Lindy, Lynn*

Lindley (English) From the pastureland *Lindly, Lindlee, Lindleigh, Lindli, Lindlie, Leland, Lindlea*

Lily

When I was pregnant, I loved the name Lily—and the fact that my daughter would be Lily of Ali, sort of like my favorite flower, lily of the valley. It may sound corny, but I felt so physically connected to her that I loved the idea that our names would also be interwined and connect us long after my pregnancy. —Ali, Montreal

Lindsay (English) From the island of linden trees; from Lincoln's wetland *Lind, Lindsea, Lindsee, Lindseigh, Lindsey, Lindsy, Linsay, Linsey*

Lisa (English) Form of Elizabeth, meaning "my God is bountiful; God's promise" *Leesa, Liesa, Lisebet, Lise, Liseta, Lisette, Liszka, Lisebeth*

Liv (Scandinavian / Latin) One who protects others / from the olive tree *Livia, Livea, Liviya, Livija, Livvy, Livy, Livya, Lyvia*

Lola (Spanish) Form of Dolores, meaning "woman of sorrow" *Lolah, Loe, Lolo*

London (English) From the capital of England *Londyn*

Lorelei (German) From the rocky cliff; in mythology, a siren who lured sailors to their deaths *Laurelei, Laurelie, Loralee, Loralei, Loralie, Loralyn*

Loretta (Italian) Form of Laura, meaning "crowned with laurel; from the laurel tree" *Laretta, Larretta, Lauretta, Laurette, Leretta, Loreta, Lorette, Lorretta*

Lorraine (French) From the kingdom of Lothair *Laraine, Larayne, Laurraine, Leraine, Lerayne, Lorain, Loraina, Loraine*

Lucy (Latin) Feminine form of Lucius; one who is illuminated *Luce, Lucetta, Lucette, Luci, Lucia, Luciana, Lucianna, Lucida, Lucille*

Luna (Latin) Of the moon *Lunah*

Lupita (Spanish) Form of Guadalupe, meaning "from the valley of wolves" *Lupe, Lupyta, Lupelina, Lupeeta, Lupieta, Lupeita, Lupeata*

Lydia (Greek) A beautiful woman from Lydia *Lidia, Lidie, Lidija, Lyda, Lydie, Lydea, Liddy, Lidiy*

Lyla (Arabic) Form of Lila, meaning "born at night / resembling a lily" *Lylah*

Lynn (English) Woman of the lake; form of Linda, meaning "one who is soft and beautiful" *Linell, Linnell, Lyn, Lynae, Lyndel, Lyndell, Lynell, Lynelle*

Lyric (French) Of the lyre; the words of a song *Lyrica, Lyricia, Lyrik, Lyrick, Lyrika, Lyricka*

M

Mackenzie (Gaelic) Daughter of a wise leader; a fiery woman; one who is fair *Mckenzie, Mackenzey, Makensie, Makenzie, M'Kenzie, McKenzie, Meckenzie, Mackenzee, Mackenzy*

Macy (French) One who wields a weapon *Macee, Macey, Maci, Macie, Maicey, Maicy, Macea, Maicea*

Maddox (English) Born into wealth and prosperity *Madox, Madoxx, Maddoxx*

Madeline (Hebrew) Woman from Magdala *Mada, Madalaina, Madaleine, Madalena, Madalene, Madelyn, Madalyn, Madelynn, Madilyn*

Madison (English) Daughter of a mighty warrior *Maddison, Madisen, Madisson, Madisyn, Madyson*

Madonna (Italian) My lady; refers to the Virgin Mary *Madonnah, Madona, Madonah*

Maeve (Irish) An intoxicating woman *Mave, Meave, Medb, Meabh*

Maggie (English) Form of Margaret, meaning "resembling a pearl" *Maggi*

Magnolia (French) Resembling the flower *Magnoliya, Magnoliah, Magnolea, Magnoleah, Magnoliyah, Magnolya, Magnolyah*

Maia (Latin / Maori) The great one; in mythology, the goddess of spring / a brave warrior *Maiah, Mya, Maja*

Maisie (Scottish) Form of Margaret, meaning "resembling a pearl" *Maisee, Maisey, Maisy, Maizie, Mazey, Mazie, Maisi, Maizi*

Makala (Hawaiian) Resembling myrtle *Makalah, Makalla, Makallah*

Makayla (Celtic / Hebrew / English) Form of Michaela, meaning "Who is like God?" *Macaela, MacKayla, Mak, Mechaela, Meeskaela, Mekea, Mekelle*

Makenna (Irish) Form of McKenna, meaning "of the Irish one" *Makennah*

Malia (Hawaiian) Form of Mary, meaning "star of the sea / from the sea of bitterness" *Maliah, Maliyah, Maleah*

Malika (Arabic) Destined to be queen *Malikah, Malyka, Maleeka, Maleika, Malieka, Maliika, Maleaka*

Marcia (Latin) Feminine form of Marcus; dedicated to Mars, the god of war *Marcena, Marcene, Marchita, Marciana, Marciane, Marcianne, Marcilyn, Marcilynn*

Marely (American) Form of Marley, meaning "of the marshy meadow"

Margaret (Greek / Persian) Resembling a pearl / the child of light *Maighread, Mairead, Mag, Maggi, Maggie, Maggy, Maiga, Malgorzata, Megan, Marwarid, Marjorie, Marged, Makareta*

Margot (French) Form of Margaret, meaning "resembling a pearl / the child of light" *Margo, Margeaux, Margaux*

Maria (Spanish) Form of Mary, meaning "star of the sea / from the sea of bitterness" *Mariah, Marialena, Marialinda, Marialisa, Maaria, Mayria, Maeria, Mariabella*

Mariah (Latin) Form of Mary, meaning "star of the sea"

Mariana (Italian / Spanish) Form of Mary, meaning "star of the sea" *Marianna*

Mariane (French) Blend of Mary, meaning "star of the sea / from the sea of bitterness," and Ann, meaning "a woman graced with God's favor" *Mariam, Mariana, Marian, Marion, Maryann, Maryanne, Maryanna, Maryane*

Marietta (French) Form of Mary, meaning "star of the sea / from the sea of bitterness" *Mariette, Maretta, Mariet, Maryetta, Maryette, Marieta*

Marika (Danish) Form of Mary, meaning "star of the sea / from the sea of bitterness"

Marilyn (English) Form of Mary, meaning "star of the sea / from the sea of bitterness" *Maralin, Maralyn, Maralynn, Marelyn, Marilee, Marilin*

Marissa (Latin) Woman of the sea *Maressa, Maricia, Marisabel, Marisha, Marisse, Maritza, Mariza, Marrissa*

Marjorie (English) Form of Margaret, meaning "resembling a pearl / the child of light" *Marcharie, Marge, Margeree, Margerie, Margery, Margey, Margi*

Marlene (German) Blend of Mary, meaning "star of the sea / from the sea of bitterness," and Magdalene, meaning "woman from Magdala" *Marlaina, Marlana, Marlane, Marlayna*

Marley (English) Of the marshy meadow *Marlee, Marleigh, Marli, Marlie, Marly*

Martha (Aramaic) Mistress of the house; in the Bible, the sister of Lazarus and Mary *Maarva, Marfa, Marhta, Mariet, Marit, Mart, Marta, Marte*

Mary (Latin / Hebrew) Star of the sea / from the sea of bitterness *Mair, Mal, Mallie, Manette, Manon, Manya, Mare, Maren, Maria, Marietta, Marika, Marilyn, Marlis, Maureen, May, Mindel, Miriam, Molly, Mia*

Maureen (Irish) Form of Mary, meaning "star of the sea / from the sea of bitterness" *Maura, Maurene, Maurianne, Maurine, Maurya, Mavra, Maure, Mo*

Mauve (French) Of the mallow plant *Mawve*

Maven (English) Having great knowledge *Mavin, Mavyn*

Mavis (French) Resembling a songbird *Mavise, Maviss, Mavisse, Mavys, Mavyss, Mavysse*

May (Latin) Born during the month of May; form of Mary, meaning "star of the sea / from the sea of bitterness" *Mae, Mai, Maelynn, Maelee, Maj, Mala, Mayana, Maye*

Maya (Indian / Hebrew) An illusion, a dream / woman of the water *Mya*

McKayla (Gaelic) A fiery woman *McKale, McKaylee, McKaleigh, McKay, McKaye, McKaela*

McKinley (English) Offspring of the fair hero

Meadow (American) From the beautiful field *Meado, Meadoe, Medow, Medowe, Medoe*

·················· **Maya** ··················

My husband wanted to name our second child after Shea Stadium, the place where we met. I thought it was a nice name for a dog, but not a child. When we chose Maya as her first name, we tried putting Shea behind it. I can't imagine a better combination now than Maya Shea. —Megan, TX

Megan (Welsh) Form of Margaret, meaning "resembling a pearl / the child of light" *Maegan, Meg, Magan, Magen, Megin, Maygan, Meagan, Meaghan, Meghan*

Melanie (Greek) A dark-skinned beauty *Malaney, Malanie, Mel, Mela, Melaina, Melaine, Melainey, Melany*

Meli (Native American) One who is bitter *Melie, Melee, Melea, Meleigh, Mely, Meley*

Melia (Hawaiian / Greek) Resembling the plumeria / of the ash tree; in mythology, a nymph *Melidice, Melitine, Meliah, Meelia, Melya*

Melika (Turkish) A great beauty *Melikah, Melicka, Melicca, Melyka, Melycka, Meleeka, Meleaka*

Melinda (Latin) One who is sweet and gentle *Melynda, Malinda, Malinde, Mallie, Mally, Malynda, Melinde, Mellinda, Mindy*

Melissa (Greek) Resembling a honeybee; in mythology, a nymph *Malissa, Mallissa, Mel, Melesa, Melessa, Melisa, Melise, Melisse*

Melody (Greek) A beautiful song *Melodee, Melodey, Melodi, Melodia, Melodie, Melodea*

Meredith (Welsh) A great ruler; protector of the sea *Maredud, Meridel, Meredithe, Meredyth, Meridith, Merridie, Meradith, Meredydd*

Mia (Israeli / Latin) Who is like God? / form of Mary, meaning "star of the sea / from the sea of bitterness" *Miah, Mea, Meah, Meya*

Michaela (Celtic / Gaelic / Hebrew / English / Irish) Feminine form of Michael, meaning "Who is like God?" *Macaela, MacKayla, Mak, Mechaela, Meeskaela, Mekea, Micaela, Mikaela*

Michelle (French) Feminine form of Michael, meaning "Who is like God?" *Machelle, Mashelle, M'chelle, Mechelle, Meechelle, Me'Shell, Meshella, Mischa*

Mikayla (English) Feminine form of Michael, meaning "Who is like God?"

Mila (Slavic) One who is industrious and hardworking *Milaia, Milaka, Milla, Milia*

Milan (Latin) From the city in Italy; one who is gracious *Milaana*

Milena (Slavic) The favored one *Mileena, Milana, Miladena, Milanka, Mlada, Mladena*

Miley (American) Form of Mili, meaning "a virtuous woman" *Milee, Mylee, Mareli*

Miliana (Latin) Feminine form of Emeliano, meaning "one who is eager and willing" *Milianah, Milianna, Miliane, Miliann, Milianne*

Mindy (English) Form of Melinda, meaning "one who is sweet and gentle" *Minda, Mindee, Mindi, Mindie, Mindey, Mindea*

Miracle (American) An act of God's hand *Mirakle, Mirakel, Myracle, Myrakle*

Miranda (Latin) Worthy of admiration *Maranda, Myranda, Randi*

Miriam (Hebrew) Form of Mary, meaning "star of the sea / from the sea of bitterness" *Mariam, Maryam, Meriam, Meryam, Mirham, Mirjam, Mirjana, Mirriam*

Molly (Irish) Form of Mary, meaning "star of the sea / from the sea of bitterness" *Moll, Mollee, Molley, Molli, Mollie, Molle, Mollea, Mali*

····························· **Miranda** ·····························

The name Miranda means "worthy of admiration" and is a Shakespeare creation. It seems to fit, as Miranda has always been the one in the family who strives for admiration by singing, acting, and telling stories and jokes. Her middle name, Elisabeth, is after my mother, who survived a double aneurysm five months before Miranda was born. —Carla, IA

Mona (Gaelic) One who is born into the nobility *Moina, Monah, Monalisa, Monalissa, Monna, Moyna, Monalysa, Monalyssa*

Monica (Greek / Latin) A solitary woman / one who advises others *Monnica, Monca, Monicka, Monika, Monike*

Monique (French) One who provides wise counsel *Moniqua, Moneeque, Moneequa, Moneeke, Moeneek, Moneaque, Moneaqua, Moneake*

Monroe (Gaelic) Woman from the river *Monrow, Monrowe, Monro*

Monserrat (Latin) From the jagged mountain *Montserrat*

Morgan (Welsh) Circling the bright sea; a sea dweller *Morgaine, Morgana, Morgance, Morgane, Morganica, Morgann, Morganne, Morgayne*

Muriel (Irish) Of the shining sea *Merial, Meriel, Merrill*

Mya (American) Form of Maya, meaning "an illusion; woman of the water" *Myah*

N

Nadia (Slavic) One who is full of hope *Nadja, Nadya, Naadiya, Nadine, Nadie, Nadiyah, Nadea, Nadija*

Nancy (English) Form of Anna, meaning "a woman graced with God's favor" *Nainsey, Nainsi, Nance, Nancee, Nancey, Nanci, Nancie, Nancsi*

Naomi (Hebrew / Japanese) One who is pleasant / a beauty above all others *Namoie, Nayomi, Naomee*

Natalia (Spanish / Latin) Form of Natalie, meaning "born on Christmas Day" *Natalya, Natalja*

Natalie (Latin) Refers to Christ's birthday; born on Christmas Day *Natala, Natalee, Nathalie, Nataline, Nataly, Natasha*

Natasha (Russian) Form of Natalie, meaning "born on Christmas Day" *Nastaliya, Nastalya, Natacha, Natascha, Natashenka, Natashia, Natasia, Natosha*

Neena (Hindi) A woman who has beautiful eyes *Neenah, Neanah, Neana, Neyna, Neynah*

Nefertiti (Egyptian) A queenly woman *Nefertari, Nefertyty, Nefertity, Nefertitie, Nefertitee, Nefertytie, Nefertitea*

Nessa (Hebrew / Greek) A miracle child / form of Agnes, meaning "one who is pure; chaste" *Nesha, Nessah, Nessia, Nessya, Nesta, Neta, Netia, Nessie*

Nevaeh (American) Child from heaven

Nicole (Greek) Feminine form of Nicholas; of the victorious people *Necole, Niccole, Nichol, Nichole, Nicholle, Nickol, Nickole, Nicol*

Noelle (French) Born at Christmastime *Noel, Noela, Noele, Noe*

Nora (English) Form of Eleanor, meaning "the shining light" *Norah, Noora, Norella, Norelle, Norissa, Norri, Norrie, Norry*

Nylah (Gaelic) Cloud or champion

O

Octavia (Latin) Feminine form of Octavius; the eighth-born child *Octaviana, Octavianne, Octavie, Octiana, Octoviana, Ottavia, Octavi, Octavy*

Odessa (Greek) Feminine form of Odysseus; one who wanders; an angry woman *Odissa, Odyssa, Odessia, Odissia, Odyssia, Odysseia*

Olivia (Latin) Feminine form of Oliver; of the olive tree; one who is peaceful *Oliviah, Oliva, Olive, Oliveea, Olivet, Olivetta, Olivette, Olivija*

························· **Olivia** ·························

We chose the name Olivia because we thought it was a beautiful name. Little did we know it would later help her learn. In kindergarten, she was always so happy to have the name with the most syllables and the most vowels to count out in class. Bonus. —Amy, KS

Olympia (Greek) From Mount Olympus; a goddess *Olympiah, Olimpe, Olimpia, Olimpiada, Olimpiana, Olypme, Olympie, Olympi*

Oona (Gaelic) Form of Agnes, meaning "one who is pure; chaste"

Opal (Sanskrit) A treasured jewel; resembling the iridescent gemstone *Opall, Opalle, Opale, Opalla, Opala, Opalina, Opaline, Opaleena*

Ophelia (Greek) One who offers help to others *Ofelia, Ofilia, OphÈlie, Ophelya, Ophilia, Ovalia, Ovelia, Opheliah*

Ophrah (Hebrew) Resembling a fawn; from the place of dust *Ofra, Ofrit, Ophra, Oprah, Orpa, Orpah, Ofrat, Ofrah*

Orion (Greek) The huntress; a constellation

Orla (Gaelic) The golden queen *Orlah, Orrla, Orrlah, Orlagh, Orlaith, Orlaithe, Orghlaith, Orghlaithe*

P

Paige (English) A young assistant *Page, Paege, Payge*

Paisley (English) Woman of the church *Paislee*

Paloma (Spanish) Dovelike *Palloma, Palomita, Palometa, Peloma, Aloma*

Pamela (English) A woman who is as sweet as honey *Pamelah, Pamella, Pammeli, Pammelie, Pameli, Pamelie, Pamelia, Pamelea*

Paris (English) Woman of the city in France *Pariss, Parisse, Parys, Paryss, Parysse*

Parker (English) The keeper of the park *Parkyr*

Parvati (Hindi) Daughter of the mountain; in Hinduism, a name for the wife of Shiva *Parvatie, Parvaty, Parvatey, Parvatee, Pauravi, Parvatea, Pauravie, Pauravy*

Patricia (English) Feminine form of Patrick; of noble descent *Patrisha, Patrycia, Patrisia, Patsy, Patti, Patty, Patrizia, Pattie, Trisha*

Paula (English) Feminine form of Paul, meaning "a petite woman" *Paulina, Pauline, Paulette, Paola, Pauleta, Pauletta, Pauli, Paulete*

Payton (English) From the warrior's village *Paton, Paeton, Paiton, Payten, Paiten*

Pearl (Latin) A precious gem of the sea *Pearla, Pearle, Pearlie, Pearly, Pearline, Pearlina, Pearli, Pearley*

Penelope (Greek) Resembling a duck; in mythology, the faithful wife of Odysseus *Peneloppe, Penelopy, Penelopey, Penelopi, Penelopie, Penelopee, Penella, Penelia, Penny*

Peony (Greek) Resembling the flower *Peoney, Peoni, Peonie, Peonee, Peonea*

Perdita (Latin) A lost woman *Perditah, Perditta, Perdy, Perdie, Perdi, Perdee, Perdea, Perdeeta*

Persephone (Greek) In mythology, the daughter of Demeter and Zeus who was abducted to the underworld *Persephoni, Persephonie, Persephony, Persephoney, Persephonee, Persefone, Persefoni, Persefonie*

Petunia (English) Resembling the flower *Petuniah, Petuniya, Petunea, Petoonia, Petounia*

Peyton (English) From the warrior's village *Peyten*

Phaedra (Greek) A bright woman; in mythology, the wife of Theseus *Phadra, Phaidra, Phedra, Phaydra, Phedre, Phaedre*

Philippa (English) Feminine form of Phillip, meaning "one who loves horses" *Phillippa, Philipa, Phillipa, Philipinna, Philippine, Phillipina, Phillipine, Pilis*

Phoebe (Greek) A bright, shining woman; in mythology, another name for the goddess of the moon *Phebe, Phoebi, Phebi, Phoebie, Phebie, Pheobe, Phoebee, Phoebea*

Phoenix (Greek) A dark-red color; in mythology, an immortal bird *Phuong, Phoenyx*

Phyllis (Greek) Of the foliage; in mythology, a girl who was turned into an almond tree *Phylis, Phillis, Philis, Phylys, Phyllida, Phylida, Phillida, Philida*

Piper (English) One who plays the flute *Pipere, Piperel, Piperell, Piperele, Piperelle, Piperela, Piperella, Pyper*

Precious (American) One who is treasured *Preshis, Preshys*

Presley (English) Of the priest's town *Presly, Preslie, Presli, Preslee*

Princess (English) A high-born daughter; born to royalty *Princessa, Princesa, Princie, Princi, Princy, Princee, Princey, Princea*

Prudence (English) One who is cautious and exercises good judgment *Prudencia, Prudensa, Prudensia, Prudentia, Predencia, Predentia, Prue, Pru*

Q

Qamra (Arabic) Of the moon *Qamrah, Qamar, Qamara, Qamrra, Qamaria, Qamrea, Qamria*

Qimat (Indian) A valuable woman *Qimate, Qimatte, Qimata, Qimatta*

Quana (Native American) One who is aromatic; sweet-smelling *Quanah, Quanna, Quannah, Quania, Quaniya, Quanniya, Quannia, Quanea*

Quincy (English) The fifth-born child *Quincey, Quinci, Quincie, Quincee, Quincia, Quinncy, Quinnci, Quyncy*

Quinn (English / Irish) Woman who is queenly *Quin, Quinne*

Quintana (Latin / English) The fifth girl / queen's lawn *Quintanah, Quinella, Quinta, Quintina, Quintanna, Quintann, Quintara, Quintona*

Quintessa (Latin) Of the essence *Quintessah, Quintesa, Quintesha, Quintisha, Quintessia, Quyntessa, Quintosha, Quinticia*

R

Rachel (Hebrew) The innocent lamb; in the Bible, Jacob's wife *Rachael, Racheal, Rachelanne, Rachelce, Rachele, Racheli, Rachell, Rachelle, Raquel*

Raina (Polish) Form of Regina, meaning "a queenly woman" *Raenah, Raene, Rainah, Raine, Rainee, Rainey, Rainelle, Rainy*

Raleigh (English) From the clearing of roe deer *Raileigh, Railey, Raley, Rawleigh, Rawley, Raly, Rali, Ralie*

Ramona (Spanish) Feminine form of Ramon; a wise protector *Ramee, Ramie, Ramoena, Ramohna, Ramonda, Ramonde, Ramonita, Ramonna*

Randi (English) Feminine form of Randall, meaning "shielded by wolves"; form of Miranda, meaning "worthy of admiration" *Randa, Randee, Randelle, Randene, Randie, Randy, Randey, Randilyn*

Raquel (Spanish) Form of Rachel, meaning "the innocent lamb" *Racquel, Racquell, Raquela, Raquelle, Roquel, Roquela, Rakel, Rakell*

Raya (Israeli) A beloved friend *Rayah*

Rayna (Hebrew / Scandinavian) One who is pure / one who provides wise counsel *Raynah, Raynee, Rayni, Rayne, Raynea, Raynie*

Reagan (Gaelic) Born into royalty; the little ruler *Raegan, Ragan, Raygan, Reganne, Regann, Regane, Reghan, Regan*

Reba (Hebrew) Form of Rebecca, meaning "one who is bound to God" *Rebah, Reeba, Rheba, Rebba, Ree, Reyba, Reaba*

Rebecca (Hebrew) One who is bound to God; in the Bible, the wife of Isaac *Rebakah, Rebbeca, Rebbecca, Rebbecka, Rebeca, Rebeccah, Rebeccea, Becky, Reba*

Reese (American) Form of Rhys, meaning "having great enthusiasm for life" *Rhyss, Rhysse, Reece, Reice, Reise, Reace, Rease, Riece*

Regina (Latin) A queenly woman *Regeena, Regena, Reggi, Reggie, Régine, Regine, Reginette, Reginia, Raina*

Remy (French) Woman from the town of Rheims *Remi, Remie, Remmy, Remmi, Remmie, Remmey, Remey*

Renée (French) One who has been reborn *Ranae, Ranay, Ranée, Renae, Renata, Renay, Renaye, René*

Reya (Spanish) A queenly woman *Reyah, Reyeh, Reye, Reyia, Reyiah, Reyea, Reyeah*

Rhea (Greek) Of the flowing stream; in mythology, the wife of Cronus and mother of gods and goddesses *Rea, Rhae, Rhaya, Rhia, Rhiah, Rhiya, Rheya*

Rhiannon (Welsh) The great and sacred queen *Rheanna, Rheanne, Rhiana, Rhiann, Rhianna, Rhiannan, Rhianon, Rhyan*

Rhonda (Welsh) Wielding a good spear *Rhondelle, Rhondene, Rhondiesha, Rhonette, Rhonnda, Ronda, Rondel, Rondelle*

Rhys (Welsh) Having great enthusiasm for life *Rhyss, Rhysse, Reece, Reese, Reice, Reise, Reace, Rease*

Rihanna (Arabic) Resembling sweet basil *Rihana*

Riley (Gaelic) From the rye clearing; a courageous woman *Reilley, Reilly, Rilee, Rileigh, Ryley, Rylee, Ryleigh, Rylie*

Rita (Greek) Precious pearl *Ritta, Reeta, Reita, Rheeta, Riet, Rieta, Ritah, Reta*

Roberta (English) Feminine form of Robert; one who is bright with fame *Robertah, Robbie, Robin*

Rochelle (French) From the little rock *Rochel, Rochele, Rochell, Rochella, Rochette, Roschella, Roschelle, Roshelle*

Ronni (English) Form of Veronica, meaning "displaying her true image" *Ronnie, Ronae, Ronay, Ronee, Ronelle, Ronette, Roni, Ronica, Ronika*

Rosalind (German / English)
Resembling a gentle horse
/ form of Rose, meaning
"resembling the beautiful
and meaningful flower" *Ros,
Rosaleen, Rosalen, Rosalin,
Rosalina, Rosalinda, Rosalinde,
Rosaline, Chalina*

Rose (Latin) Resembling the
beautiful and meaningful
flower *Rosa, Rosie, Rosalind,
Rosalyn*

Roseanne (English)
Resembling the graceful
rose *Ranna, Rosana, Rosanagh,
Rosanna, Rosannah, Rosanne,
Roseann, Roseanna*

Rosemary (Latin / English)
The dew of the sea / resem-
bling a bitter rose *Rosemaree,
Rosemarey, Rosemaria,
Rosemarie, Rosmarie, Rozmary,
Rosamaria, Rosamarie*

Rowan (Gaelic) Of the
redberry tree *Rowann, Rowane,
Rowanne, Rowana, Rowanna*

Rowena (Welsh / German)
One who is fair and slender
/ having much fame and
happiness *Rhowena, Roweena,
Roweina, Rowenna, Rowina,
Rowinna, Rhonwen, Rhonwyn*

Ruby (English) As precious as
the red gemstone *Rubee, Rubi,
Rubie, Rubyna, Rubea*

Rue (English, German) A
medicinal herb *Ru, Larue*

Ruth (Hebrew) A beloved
companion *Ruthe, Ruthelle,
Ruthellen, Ruthetta, Ruthi, Ruthie,
Ruthina, Ruthine*

Ryder (American) An accom-
plished horsewoman *Rider*

Rylee (American) Form of
Riley, meaning "from the
rye clearing; a courageous
woman"

S

Sabrina (English) A legendary princess *Sabrinah, Sabrinna, Sabreena, Sabriena, Sabreina, Sabryna, Sabrine, Sabryne, Cabrina, Zabrina*

Sadie (English) Form of Sarah, meaning "a princess; lady" *Sadi, Sady, Sadey, Sadee, Saddi, Saddee, Sadiey, Sadye*

Sailor (American) One who sails the seas *Sailer, Sailar, Saylor, Sayler, Saylar, Saelor, Saeler, Saelar*

Samantha (Aramaic) One who listens well *Samanthah, Samanthia, Samanthea, Samantheya, Samanath, Samanatha, Samana, Samanitha*

Samone (Hebrew) Form of Simone, meaning "one who listens well" *Samoan, Samoane, Samon, Samona, Samonia*

Sandra (Greek) Form of Alexandra, meaning "a helper and defender of mankind" *Sandrah, Sandrine, Sandy, Sandi, Sandie, Sandey, Sandee, Sanda, Sandrica*

Sandrine (Greek) Form of Alexandra, meaning "a helper and defender of mankind" *Sandrin, Sandreana, Sandreanah, Sandreane, Sandreen, Sandreena, Sandreenah, Sandreene*

Santana (Spanish) A saintly woman *Santa, Santah, Santania, Santaniah, Santaniata, Santena, Santenah, Santenna*

Saoirse (Gaelic) An independent woman; having freedom *Saoyrse*

Sasha (Russian) Form of Alexandra, meaning "a helper and defender of mankind" *Sascha, Sashenka, Saskia*

Savannah (English) From the open grassy plain *Savanna, Savana, Savanne, Savann, Savane, Savanneh*

Scarlett (English) Vibrant red color; a vivacious woman *Scarlet, Scarlette, Skarlet*

Selene (Greek) Of the moon *Celina, Sela, Selena, Selina, Zalina*

Serafina (Latin) A seraph; a heavenly, winged angel *Serafinah, Serafine, Seraphina, Serefina, Seraphine, Sera*

Serena (Latin) Having a peaceful disposition *Serenah, Serene, Sereena, Seryna, Serenity, Serenitie, Serenitee, Serepta, Cerina, Xerena*

Serenity (Latin) Peaceful

Shakira (Arabic) Feminine form of Shakir; grateful; thankful *Shakirah, Shakiera, Shaakira, Shakeira, Shakyra, Shakeyra, Shakura, Shakirra*

Shannon (Gaelic) Having ancient wisdom; river name *Shanon, Shannen, Shannan, Shannin, Shanna, Shannae, Shannun, Shannyn*

Sheila (Irish) Form of Cecilia, meaning "one who is blind" *Sheilah, Sheelagh, Shelagh, Shiela, Shyla, Selia, Sighle, Sheiletta*

Sharon (Hebrew) From the plains; a flowering shrub *Sharron, Sharone, Sharona, Shari, Sharis, Sharne, Sherine, Sharun*

Shelby (English) From the willow farm *Shelbi, Shelbey, Shelbie, Shelbee, Shelbye, Shelbea*

Shayla (Irish) Of the fairy palace; form of Shai, meaning "a gift of God" *Shaylah, Shaylagh, Shaylain, Shaylan, Shaylea, Shayleah, Shaylla, Sheyla*

Sheridan (Gaelic) One who is wild and untamed; a searcher *Sheridann, Sheridanne, Sherydan, Sherridan, Sheriden, Sheridon, Sherrerd, Sherida*

Sibyl (English) A prophetess; a seer *Sybil, Sibyla, Sybella, Sibil, Sibella, Sibilla, Sibley, Sibylla*

Shaylee (Gaelic) From the fairy palace; a fairy princess *Shalee, Shayleigh, Shailee, Shaileigh, Shaelee, Shaeleigh, Shayli, Shaylie*

Sienna (Italian) Woman with reddish-brown hair *Siena, Siennya, Sienya, Syenna, Syinna*

Sierra (Spanish) From the jagged mountain range *Siera, Syerra, Syera, Seyera, Seeara*

Simone (French) One who listens well *Sim, Simonie, Symone, Samone*

Skylar (English) One who is learned, a scholar *Skylare, Skylarr, Skyler, Skylor, Skylir*

Sloane (Irish) A strong protector; a woman warrior *Sloan, Slone*

Sophia (Greek) Form of Sophie, meaning "great wisdom and foresight" *Sofia, Sofiya*

Sophie (Greek) Great wisdom and foresight *Sophia, Sofiya, Sofie, Sofia, Sofi, Sofiyko, Sofronia, Sophronia, Zofia*

Sparrow (English) Resembling a small songbird *Sparro, Sparroe, Sparo, Sparow, Sparowe, Sparoe*

····· **Sloane** ·····

My husband and I named our girls Cameron and Sloane... because we're obsessed with the movie *Ferris Bueller's Day Off*! —Brenda, MD

························· **Stella** ·························

We chose Stella because it is classic and there aren't many Stellas out there. And it's a beautiful-sounding name. Unfortunately, every time we tell it to people, inevitably someone does their best Marlon Brando impression: "Stella!!! Pick up those toys!" But I don't care; it's still a great name.
—Sarah, IL

Stacey (English) Form of Anastasia, meaning "one who shall rise again" *Stacy, Staci, Stacie, Stacee, Stacia, Stasia, Stasy, Stasey*

Stella (English) Star of the sea *Stela, Stelle, Stele, Stellah, Stelah*

Stephanie (Greek) Feminine form of Stephen, meaning "crowned with garland" *Stephani, Stephany, Stephaney, Stephanee, Stephene, Stephana, Stefanie, Stefani*

Summer (American) Refers to the season; born in summer *Sommer, Sumer, Somer, Somers*

Susannah (Hebrew) White lily *Susanna, Susanne, Susana, Susane, Susan, Suzanna, Suzannah, Suzanne, Shoshana, Huhana*

Sydney (English) Of the wide meadow *Sydny, Sydni, Sydnie, Sydnea, Sydnee, Sidney, Sidne, Sidnee*

T

Tabitha (Greek) Resembling a gazelle; known for beauty and grace *Tabithah, Tabbitha, Tabetha, Tabbetha, Tabatha, Tabbatha, Tabotha, Tabbotha*

Talia (Hebrew / Greek) Morning dew from heaven / blooming *Taliah, Talea, Taleah, Taleya, Tallia, Talieya, Taleea, Taleia*

Tara (Gaelic / Indian) Of the tower; rocky hill / star; in mythology, an astral goddess *Tarah, Tarra, Tayra, Taraea, Tarai, Taralee, Tarali, Taraya*

Tatum (English) Bringer of joy; spirited *Tatom, Tatim, Tatem, Tatam, Tatym*

Taylor (English) Cutter of cloth; one who alters garments *Tailor, Taylore, Taylar, Tayler, Talour, Taylre, Tailore, Tailar*

Teagan (Gaelic) One who is attractive *Teegan*

Teresa (Greek) A harvester *Theresa, Theresah, Theresia, Therese, Thera, Tresa, Tressa, Tressam, Reese, Reza*

Tessa (Greek) Form of Teresa, meaning "a harvester"

Thea (Greek) A goddess; in mythology, the mother of the sun, moon, and dawn *Thia, Thya, Theia*

Thelma (Greek) One who is ambitious and willful *Thelmah, Telma, Thelmai, Thelmia, Thelmalina*

Tia (Spanish / Greek) An aunt / daughter born to royalty *Tiah, Tea, Teah, Tiana, Teea, Tya, Teeya, Tiia*

Tiegan (Aztec) A little princess in a big valley *Tiegann, Tieganne*

Tiffany (Greek) Lasting love *Tiffaney, Tiffani, Tiffanie, Tiffanee, Tifany, Tifaney, Tifanee, Tifani*

Tina (English) From the river; also shortened form of names ending in -tina *Tinah, Teena, Tena, Teyna, Tyna, Tinna, Teana*

Tory (American) Form of Victoria, meaning "victorious woman; winner; conqueror" *Torry, Torey, Tori, Torie, Torree, Tauri, Torye, Toya*

Trinity (Latin) The holy three *Trinitey, Triniti, Trinitie, Trinitee, Trynity, Trynitey, Tryniti, Trynitie*

Trisha (Latin) Form of Patricia, meaning "of noble descent" *Trishah, Trishia, Tricia, Trish, Trissa, Trisa*

Trishna (Polish) In mythology, the goddess of the deceased, protector of graves *Trishnah, Trishnia, Trishniah, Trishnea, Trishneah, Trishniya, Trishniyah, Trishnya*

Trudy (German) Form of Gertrude, meaning "adored warrior" *Trudey, Trudi, Trudie, Trude, Trudye, Trudee, Truda, Trudia*

Tula (Hindi) Balance; a sign of the zodiac *Tulah, Tulla, Tullah*

U

Ualani (Hawaiian) Of the heavenly rain *Ualanie, Ualany, Ualaney, Ualanee, Ualanea, Ualania, Ualana*

Udele (English) One who is wealthy; prosperous *Udelle, Udela, Udella, Udelah, Udellah, Uda, Udah*

Ulla (German) A willful woman *Ullah, Ullaa, Ullai, Ullae*

Uma (Hindi) Mother; in mythology, the goddess of beauty and sunlight *Umah, Umma*

Unity (American) Woman who upholds oneness; togetherness *Unitey, Unitie, Uniti, Unitee, Unitea, Unyty, Unytey, Unytie*

V

Valencia (Spanish) One who is powerful; strong; from the city of Valencia *Valenciah, Valyncia, Valencya, Valenzia, Valancia, Valenica, Valanca, Valecia*

Valentina (Latin) One who is vigorous and healthy *Valentinah, Valentine, Valenteena, Valenteana, Valentena, Valentyna, Valantina, Valentyne*

Valeria (Latin) Form of Valerie, meaning "strong and valiant" *Valara, Valera, Valaria, Valeriana, Veleria, Valora*

Valerie (Latin) Feminine form of Valerius; strong and valiant *Valeri, Valeree, Valerey, Valery, Valarie, Valari, Vallcry*

Vanessa (Greek) Resembling a butterfly *Vanessah, Vanesa, Vannesa, Vannessa, Vanassa, Vanasa, Vanessia, Vanysa, Yanessa*

Veronica (Latin) Displaying her true image *Veronicah, Veronic, Veronicca, Veronicka, Veronika, Veronicha, Veronique, Veranique, Ronni*

Victoria (Latin) Victorious woman; winner; conqueror *Victoriah, Victorea, Victoreah, Victorya, Victorria, Victoriya, Vyctoria, Victorine, Tory*

Violet (French) Resembling the purplish-blue flower *Violett, Violette, Violete, Vyolet, Vyolett, Vyolette, Vyolete, Violeta*

Viveka (German) Little woman of the strong fortress *Vivekah, Vivecka, Vyveka, Viveca, Vyveca, Vivecca, Vivika, Vivieka*

Virginia (Latin) One who is chaste; virginal; from the state of Virginia *Virginiah, Virginnia, Virgenya, Virgenia, Virgeenia, Virgeena, Virgena, Ginny*

Vivian (Latin) Lively woman *Viv, Vivi, Vivienne, Bibiana*

W

Walker (English) Walker of the forests *Wallker, Walkher*

Wendy (Welsh) Form of Gwendolyn, meaning "one who is fair; of the white ring" *Wendi, Wendie, Wendee, Wendey, Wenda, Wendia, Wendea, Wendya*

Wesley (English) From the western meadow *Wesly, Weslie, Wesli, Weslee, Weslia, Wesleigh, Weslea, Weslei*

Whitney (English) From the white island *Whitny, Whitnie, Whitni, Whitnee, Whittney, Whitneigh, Whytny, Whytney*

Wilhelmina (German) Feminine form of Wilhelm; determined protector *Wilhelminah, Wylhelmina, Wylhelmyna, Willemina, Wilhelmine, Wilhemina, Wilhemine, Helma, Ilma*

···························· **Whitney** ····························

We named our girl Whitney Renee. We were looking for a name that was unique and familiar at the same time. —Dawn & Chad, IL

Willa (English) Feminine version of William, meaning "protector" *Willah, Wylla*

Willow (English) One who is hoped for; desired *Willo, Willough*

Wren (English) Resembling a small songbird *Wrenn, Wrene, Wrena, Wrenie, Wrenee, Wreney, Wrenny, Wrenna*

Xerena (Latin) Form of Serena, meaning "having a peaceful disposition" *Xerenah, Xerene, Xeren, Xereena, Xeryna, Xereene, Xerenna*

Xhosa (African) Leader of a nation *Xosa, Xhose, Xhosia, Xhosah, Xosah*

Xiang (Chinese) Having a nice fragrance *Xyang, Xeang, Xhiang, Xhyang, Xheang*

Xiao Hong (Chinese) Of the morning rainbow

Xin Qian (Chinese) Happy and beautiful woman

Xirena (Greek) Form of Sirena, meaning "enchantress" *Xirenah, Xireena, Xirina, Xirene, Xyrena, Xyreena, Xyrina, Xyryna*

Y

Yana (Hebrew) He answers
Yanna, Yaan, Yanah, Yannah

Yara (Brazilian) In mythology, the goddess of the river; a mermaid *Yarah, Yarrah, Yarra*

Yareli (American) The Lord is my light *Yarelie, Yareley, Yarelee, Yarely, Yaresly, Yarelea, Yareleah*

Yaretzi (Spanish) Always beloved *Yaretza, Yaretzie, Yarezita*

Yasmine (Persian) Resembling the jasmine flower *Yasmin, Yasmene, Yasmeen, Yasmeene, Yasmen, Yasemin, Yasemeen, Yasmyn*

Ynes (French) Form of Agnes, meaning "one who is pure; chaste" *Ynez, Ynesita*

Yolanda (Greek) Resembling the violet flower *Yola, Yolana, Yolandah, Colanda*

Yvonne (French) Young archer *Yvone, Vonne, Vonna*

Z

Zabrina (American) Form of Sabrina, meaning "a legendary princess" *Zabreena, Zabrinah, Zabrinna, Zabryna, Zabryne, Zabrynya, Zabreana, Zabreane*

Zahra (Arabic / Swahili) White-skinned / flowerlike *Zahrah, Zahraa, Zahre, Zahreh, Zahara, Zaharra, Zahera, Zahira*

Zariah (Russian / Slavic) Born at sunrise *Zarya, Zaria, Zaryah*

Zaylee (English) A heavenly woman *Zayleigh, Zayli, Zaylie, Zaylea, Zayleah, Zayley, Zayly, Zalee*

Zephyr (Greek) Of the west wind *Zephyra, Zephira, Zephria, Zephra, Zephyer, Zefiryn, Zefiryna, Zefyrin*

Ziona (Hebrew) One who symbolizes goodness *Zionah, Zyona, Zyonah*

Zoe (Greek) A life-giving woman; alive *Zoee, Zowey, Zowie, Zowe, Zoelie, Zoeline, Zoelle, Zoey*

Zuri (Swahili / French) A beauty / lovely and white *Zurie, Zurey, Zuria, Zuriaa, Zury, Zuree, Zurya, Zurisha*

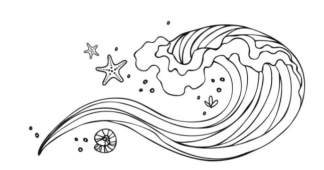

The Top 1,000

N eed some more options? Here are the recent top 1,000 girls names in the United States according to the Social Security Administration:

Aadhya	Adelaide	Aisha	Alejandra
Aaliyah	Adele	Aitana	Alena
Abby	Adelina	Aiyana	Alessandra
Abigail	Adeline	Alaia	Alessia
Abril	Adelyn	Alaina	Alexa
Ada	Adelynn	Alana	Alexandra
Adaline	Adilynn	Alani	Alexandria
Adalyn	Adley	Alanna	Alexia
Adalynn	Adriana	Alannah	Alexis
Addilyn	Adrianna	Alaya	Alia
Addilynn	Adrienne	Alayah	Aliana
Addison	Ailani	Alayna	Alice
Addisyn	Aileen	Aleah	Alicia
Addyson	Ainsley	Aleena	Alina

Alisa	Amelie	Aniya	Ariella
Alisha	Amia	Aniyah	Arielle
Alison	Amina	Anna	Ariya
Alivia	Aminah	Annabel	Ariyah
Aliya	Amira	Annabella	Armani
Aliyah	Amirah	Annabelle	Arya
Aliza	Amiya	Annalee	Aryanna
Allie	Amiyah	Annalise	Ashley
Allison	Amora	Anne	Ashlyn
Allyson	Amy	Annie	Ashlynn
Alma	Ana	Annika	Aspen
Alondra	Anabelle	Ansley	Astrid
Alora	Anahi	Antonella	Athena
Alyson	Analia	Anya	Aubree
Alyssa	Anastasia	April	Aubrey
Amalia	Anaya	Arabella	Aubrie
Amanda	Andi	Aranza	Aubriella
Amani	Andrea	Arely	Aubrielle
Amara	Angel	Ari	Audrey
Amari	Angela	Aria	Audrina
Amaris	Angelica	Ariadne	Aurelia
Amaya	Angelina	Ariah	Aurora
Amayah	Angelique	Ariana	Autumn
Amber	Angie	Arianna	Ava
Amelia	Anika	Ariel	Avah

Avalyn	Blaire	Brynn	Caylee
Avalynn	Blake	Cadence	Cecelia
Averi	Blakely	Cali	Cecilia
Averie	Bonnie	Callie	Celeste
Avery	Braelyn	Calliope	Celia
Aviana	Braelynn	Cameron	Celine
Avianna	Braylee	Camila	Chana
Aya	Breanna	Camilla	Chanel
Ayla	Brenda	Camille	Charlee
Ayleen	Brenna	Camryn	Charleigh
Aylin	Bria	Cara	Charley
Azalea	Briana	Carla	Charli
Azariah	Brianna	Carlee	Charlie
Bailee	Briar	Carly	Charlotte
Bailey	Bridget	Carmen	Chaya
Barbara	Briella	Carolina	Chelsea
Baylee	Brielle	Caroline	Cheyenne
Beatrice	Brinley	Carolyn	Chloe
Belen	Bristol	Carter	Christina
Bella	Brittany	Casey	Christine
Belle	Brooke	Cassandra	Claire
Bethany	Brooklyn	Cassidy	Clara
Bexley	Brooklynn	Cataleya	Clare
Bianca	Brylee	Catalina	Clarissa
Blair	Brynlee	Catherine	Claudia

Clementine	Delaney	Ella	Emilia
Colette	Delilah	Elle	Emily
Collins	Demi	Ellen	Emma
Cora	Desiree	Elliana	Emmaline
Coraline	Destiny	Ellianna	Emmalyn
Corinne	Diana	Ellie	Emmalynn
Courtney	Dorothy	Elliot	Emmeline
Crystal	Dream	Elliott	Emmie
Cynthia	Dulce	Ellis	Emmy
Dahlia	Dylan	Ellison	Emory
Daisy	Eden	Eloise	Ensley
Dakota	Edith	Elora	Erica
Dalary	Egypt	Elsa	Erika
Daleyza	Eileen	Elsie	Erin
Dallas	Elaina	Elyse	Esme
Dana	Elaine	Ember	Esmeralda
Danica	Eleanor	Emberly	Esperanza
Daniela	Elena	Emelia	Estella
Daniella	Eliana	Emely	Estelle
Danielle	Elianna	Emerald	Esther
Danna	Elisa	Emerie	Estrella
Daphne	Elisabeth	Emerson	Eva
Davina	Elise	Emersyn	Evalyn
Dayana	Eliza	Emery	Evangeline
Deborah	Elizabeth	Emilee	Eve

Evelyn	Genevieve	Hallie	Hope
Evelynn	Georgia	Hana	Hunter
Everlee	Gia	Hanna	Iliana
Everleigh	Giana	Hannah	Imani
Everly	Gianna	Harlee	India
Evie	Giovanna	Harleigh	Ingrid
Faith	Giselle	Harley	Irene
Fatima	Giuliana	Harlow	Iris
Faye	Gloria	Harmoni	Isabel
Felicity	Grace	Harmony	Isabela
Fernanda	Gracelyn	Harper	Isabella
Finley	Gracelynn	Hattie	Isabelle
Fiona	Gracie	Haven	Isla
Florence	Greta	Hayden	Itzayana
Frances	Guadalupe	Haylee	Itzel
Francesca	Gwen	Hayley	Ivanna
Frankie	Gwendolyn	Hazel	Ivory
Freya	Hadassah	Heaven	Ivy
Frida	Hadlee	Heavenly	Izabella
Gabriela	Hadleigh	Heidi	Jacqueline
Gabriella	Hadley	Helen	Jada
Gabrielle	Hailee	Helena	Jade
Galilea	Hailey	Henley	Jaelyn
Gemma	Haley	Holland	Jaelynn
Genesis	Halle	Holly	Jaliyah

Jamie	Jessica	Julie	Kamryn
Jana	Jessie	Juliet	Kara
Jane	Jewel	Julieta	Karen
Janelle	Jillian	Juliette	Karina
Janessa	Jimena	Julissa	Karla
Janiyah	Joanna	June	Karlee
Jasmine	Jocelyn	Juniper	Karlie
Jaycee	Joelle	Jurnee	Karsyn
Jayda	Johanna	Justice	Karter
Jayde	Jolene	Kadence	Kassandra
Jayden	Jolie	Kaelyn	Kassidy
Jayla	Jordan	Kai	Katalina
Jaylah	Jordyn	Kaia	Kate
Jaylee	Joselyn	Kailani	Katelyn
Jayleen	Josephine	Kailee	Katherine
Jaylene	Josie	Kailey	Kathleen
Jazlyn	Joslyn	Kailyn	Kathryn
Jazlynn	Journee	Kairi	Katie
Jazmin	Journey	Kaitlyn	Kaya
Jazmine	Joy	Kaiya	Kaydence
Jemma	Joyce	Kalani	Kayla
Jenna	Judith	Kali	Kaylani
Jennifer	Julia	Kaliyah	Kaylee
Jenny	Juliana	Kallie	Kayleigh
Jessa	Julianna	Kamila	Kaylie

Kaylin	Kinslee	Laylah	Lilith
Kehlani	Kinsley	Lea	Lillian
Keira	Kira	Leah	Lilliana
Kelly	Kora	Leanna	Lillianna
Kelsey	Kori	Legacy	Lillie
Kendall	Kristina	Leia	Lilly
Kendra	Kyla	Leighton	Lily
Kenia	Kylee	Leila	Lilyana
Kenley	Kyleigh	Leilani	Lina
Kenna	Kylie	Lena	Linda
Kennedi	Kynlee	Lennon	Lindsey
Kennedy	Kyra	Lennox	Lisa
Kensley	Lacey	Leona	Liv
Kenya	Laila	Leslie	Livia
Kenzie	Lailah	Lexi	Lizbeth
Keyla	Lainey	Lexie	Logan
Khaleesi	Lana	Leyla	Lola
Khloe	Landry	Lia	London
Kiana	Laney	Liana	Londyn
Kiara	Lara	Liberty	Lorelai
Kiera	Laura	Lila	Lorelei
Kimber	Laurel	Lilah	Louisa
Kimberly	Lauren	Lilian	Louise
Kimora	Lauryn	Liliana	Lucia
Kinley	Layla	Lilianna	Luciana

Lucille	Madisyn	Mariam	Melania
Lucy	Mae	Mariana	Melanie
Luella	Maeve	Marianna	Melany
Luna	Magdalena	Marie	Melina
Lyanna	Maggie	Marilyn	Melissa
Lydia	Magnolia	Marina	Melody
Lyla	Maia	Marissa	Mercy
Lylah	Maisie	Marjorie	Meredith
Lyra	Makayla	Marlee	Mia
Lyric	Makenna	Marleigh	Miah
Mabel	Makenzie	Marley	Micah
Maci	Malani	Marlowe	Michaela
Macie	Malaya	Martha	Michelle
Mackenzie	Malaysia	Mary	Mikaela
Macy	Maleah	Maryam	Mikayla
Madalyn	Malia	Matilda	Mila
Madalynn	Maliah	Mavis	Milan
Maddison	Maliyah	Maxine	Milana
Madeleine	Mallory	Maya	Milani
Madeline	Mara	Mckenna	Milena
Madelyn	Maren	Mckenzie	Miley
Madelynn	Margaret	Mckinley	Millie
Madilyn	Margot	Meadow	Mina
Madilynn	Maria	Megan	Mira
Madison	Mariah	Meilani	Miracle

Miranda	Nayeli	Paige	Quinn
Miriam	Nevaeh	Paislee	Rachel
Miya	Nia	Paisleigh	Raegan
Molly	Nicole	Paisley	Raelyn
Monica	Nina	Paityn	Raelynn
Monroe	Noa	Paloma	Raina
Monserrat	Noelle	Paola	Ramona
Morgan	Noemi	Paris	Raquel
Mya	Nola	Parker	Raven
Myah	Noor	Patricia	Raylee
Myla	Nora	Paula	Rayna
Mylah	Norah	Paulina	Rayne
Myra	Nova	Payton	Reagan
Nadia	Novalee	Pearl	Rebecca
Nala	Nyla	Penelope	Rebekah
Nalani	Nylah	Penny	Reese
Nancy	Oaklee	Perla	Regina
Naomi	Oakley	Peyton	Reign
Natalia	Oaklyn	Phoebe	Reina
Natalie	Oaklynn	Phoenix	Remi
Nataly	Octavia	Piper	Remington
Natasha	Olive	Poppy	Remy
Nathalia	Olivia	Presley	Renata
Nathalie	Opal	Princess	Renee
Naya	Ophelia	Priscilla	Reyna

Rhea	Saanvi	Selena	Summer
Riley	Sabrina	Selene	Sunny
River	Sadie	Serena	Susan
Rivka	Sage	Serenity	Sutton
Riya	Saige	Shelby	Sydney
Romina	Salma	Shiloh	Sylvia
Rory	Samantha	Siena	Sylvie
Rosa	Samara	Sienna	Talia
Rosalie	Samira	Sierra	Taliyah
Rosalyn	Sandra	Simone	Tara
Rose	Saoirse	Sky	Tatiana
Roselyn	Sara	Skye	Tatum
Rosemary	Sarah	Skyla	Taylor
Rosie	Sarai	Skylar	Teagan
Rowan	Sariah	Skyler	Tegan
Royal	Sariyah	Sloan	Tenley
Royalty	Sasha	Sloane	Teresa
Ruby	Savanna	Sofia	Tessa
Ruth	Savannah	Sonia	Thalia
Ryan	Sawyer	Sophia	Thea
Ryann	Saylor	Sophie	Tiana
Rylan	Scarlet	Spencer	Tiffany
Rylee	Scarlett	Stella	Tinley
Ryleigh	Scarlette	Stephanie	Tinsley
Rylie	Selah	Stevie	Tori

Treasure	Vienna	Wynter	Zaria
Trinity	Violet	Ximena	Zariah
Vada	Virginia	Xiomara	Zariyah
Valentina	Vivian	Yamileth	Zaylee
Valeria	Viviana	Yara	Zelda
Valerie	Vivienne	Yareli	Zendaya
Vanessa	Whitney	Yaretzi	Zion
Veda	Willa	Zahra	Zoe
Vera	Willow	Zainab	Zoey
Veronica	Winter	Zaniyah	Zoie
Victoria	Wren	Zara	Zuri

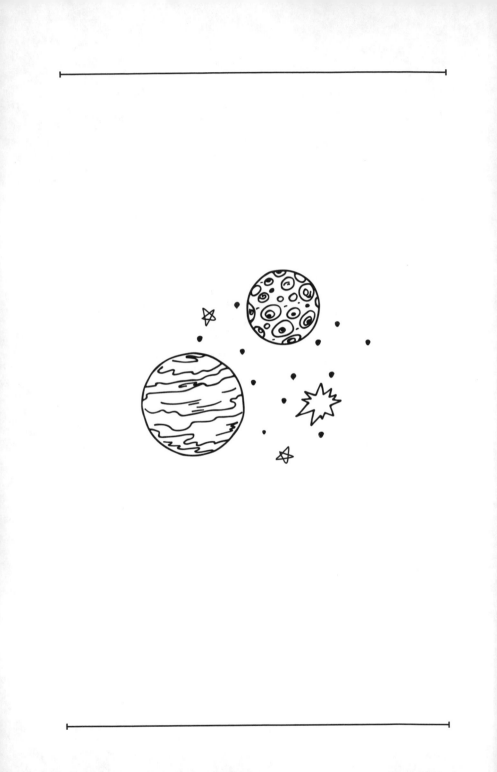

My Favorite Names ♡

....
....
....
....
....
....
....
....
....
....
....
....
....
....
....
....
....
....
....
....
....
....
....
....

My Favorite Names ♡

My Favorite Names ♡

My Favorite Names ♡

My Favorite Names ♡

....
....
....
....
....
....
....
....
....
....
....
....
....
....
....
....
....
....
....
....
....
....
....

My Favorite Names ♡

My Favorite Names ♡

My Favorite Names ♡

....

....

....

....

....

....

....

....

....

....

....

....

....

....

....

....

....

....

....

....

....

....

My Favorite Names ♡

My Favorite Names ♡

My Favorite Names ♡